THE Men'sHealth LITTLE BOOK OF EXERCISES

MACMILLAN

First published in the USA in 2014 by Rodale Inc.

First published in the UK 2015 by Macmillan
an imprint of Pan Macmillan, a division of Macmillan Publishers Limited
Pan Macmillan, 20 New Wharf Road, London N1 9RR
Basingstoke and Oxford
Associated companies throughout the world
www.panmacmillan.com

ISBN 978-1-4472-9072-8

Book design by George Karabotsos with John Seeger Gilman
Cover design by Joe Heroun

Photo editor: Mark Haddad

All photography by Beth Bischoff
Cover makeup artist: Lynn Lamorte at Vivian Artists
Exercise footwear and apparel provided by Nike, Adidas and Under Armour
Anatomy illustrations by bartleby.com, except Gluteus Maximus illustration by Kurt Walters

Printed and bound in Italy by Printer Trento

This book is intended as a reference volume only, not as a medical manual. The information
given here is designed to help you make informed decisions about your health. It is not intended
as a substitute for any treatment that you may have been prescribed by your doctor. If you
suspect that you have a medical problem, we urge you to seek competent medical help.

The information in this book is meant to supplement, not replace, proper exercise training.
All forms of exercise pose some inherent risks. The editor and publisher advise readers to take full
responsibility for their safety and know their limits. Before practicing the exercises in this book be
sure that your equipment is well maintained, and do not take risks beyond your level of experience,
aptitude, training and fitness. The exercise programme in this book is not intended as a substitute
for any exercise routine that may have been prescribed by your doctor. As with all exercise
programmes, you should get your doctor's approval before beginning.

Visit **www.panmacmillan.com** to read more about all our books
and to buy them. You will also find features, author interviews and
news of any author events, and you can sign up for e-newsletters
so that you're always first to hear about our new releases.

Contents

Introduction
Your New Body Starts Here

How to Use This Book to Get Big and Strong

This book is custom-made for you. Whether you want to lose flab hanging over your belt, build large, well-defined muscles, or get your body into prime shape for your athletic endeavors (maybe some combo of all three?), *The Men's Health Little Book of Exercises* is full of perfect tools to get you there.

Based on the bestselling *Men's Health Big Book of Exercises,* this new volume is even more practical and easy to use. It's brief, it's a really smart reference guide to some of the best strength-training, muscle-building, fat-burning resistance exercises you can do, and it's packaged in a handy format that you can easily take with you wherever you go to do this important work.

The pictures and captions inside provide great instruction for moves you may not have committed to memory, and they are big enough that you can check your form at a glance, which is an essential part of getting the most benefit from an exercise.

On the pages that follow, you'll find chapters broken down by main muscle groups, starting with chest exercises. In each chapter, you'll learn proper execution of "Main Move" exercises followed by variations on those moves. These changeups challenge your muscles in different ways, so they're terrific to use to sculpt well-defined muscles as well as build out-of-this-world functional strength. (*Psst,* they'll also keep your workouts fresh and your muscles guessing!) There's also a chapter on total-body exercises that you'll want to try for a highly effective fat-burning metabolic workout, especially when your time is tight.

After the instructional exercise chapters comes a large chapter called "The Best Workouts for Everything," starting on page 200. No matter what your goal, you'll find innovative workouts to challenge your body like never before so you can build the physique you've never experienced before but have always dreamed of.

Work hard and you will be rewarded. Now, have at it!

Chest

A muscular chest is powerful. It increases your presence in the boardroom, wins her over in the bedroom, and intimidates on the playing field. So it's no surprise that guys have an affinity for exercises that build their chests. Your pecs, after all, are the most prominent muscle you see in your bathroom mirror. And who doesn't want to improve that image?

What's more, if you stop lifting weights, your chest is one of the first muscle groups that will atrophy. That's because you rarely stress these muscles in daily activities. Think about it: How often in real life do you have to push heavy weights away from your chest? Keep in mind that losing muscle slows your metabolism—which means regularly training your chest also helps you fight belly fat.

The Bonus Benefits of a Bigger Chest

More power: Stronger chest muscles make it easier to push off opponents in any contact sport, whether your game is football, basketball, martial arts, or hockey.

A stronger swing: Forehand strokes in tennis and sidearm throws in baseball rely on powerful chest muscles for velocity, in addition to your core musculature.

A knockout punch: The chest's primary objective is to move the arms forward, so developing pectoral strength helps you deliver more energy into your target.

Meet Your Muscles

Pectoralis Major

Your main chest muscle is the pectoralis major [1]. Its job: to pull your upper arms toward the middle of your body. Think about that in terms of a bench press. As you push the bar away from your torso, your upper arms move closer to your chest as they straighten. This is because your pectoralis major attaches to the inside of your upper arm bone. So when your pectorals contract, the muscle fibers shorten, pulling your upper arms toward the muscles' origin, your mid-chest.

This is why exercises such as pushups and bench presses are the best way to make your pecs pop. By holding a weight in your hands when you do a bench press, for instance, you increase the weight of your upper arms, which forces your pectoral muscles to contract harder. The end result: a bigger, stronger chest.

The sternal portion of the muscle is collectively considered to be your lower chest.

The muscle fibers that make up the clavicular portion form what many call the upper chest.

The fibers of your pectoralis major originate at three places on your chest: your collarbone [2], your breastbone [3], and your ribs [4], just below your breastbone.

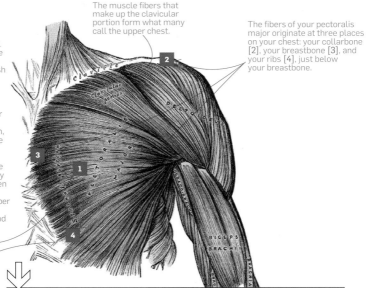

Pectoralis Minor

The pectoralis minor [5] is a thin, triangular muscle that lies beneath your pectoralis major. It starts at your third, fourth, and fifth ribs and attaches near your shoulder joint. Although this muscle is technically a "chest muscle," its main duty is to assist in pulling your shoulders forward—an action that occurs in back exercises such as the dumbbell pullover.

Chest |

In this chapter, you'll find 48 exercises that target the muscles of your chest. Throughout, you'll notice that certain exercises have been designated as a Main Move. Master this basic version of a movement, and you'll be able to do all of its variations with flawless form.

PUSHUPS

These exercises target your pectoralis major. However, they also hit your front deltoids and triceps, since these muscles assist in just about every version of the movements. What's more, your rotator, trapezius, serratus anterior, and abdominals all contract to keep your shoulders, core, and hips stable as you perform the moves.

MAIN MOVE
Pushup

- Get down on all fours and place your hands on the floor so that they're slightly wider than and in line with your shoulders.

Squeeze your glutes and hold them that way for the entire movement. This helps keep your hips stable and in line with your upper body.

Your arms should be straight.

Your body should form a straight line from your ankles to your head.

Straighten your legs, with your weight on your toes.

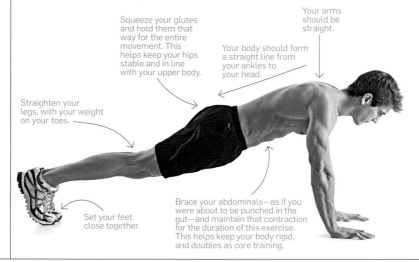

Set your feet close together.

Brace your abdominals—as if you were about to be punched in the gut—and maintain that contraction for the duration of this exercise. This helps keep your body rigid, and doubles as core training.

75

Percent of your body weight you lift when you do a standard pushup, according to research by the National Strength and Conditioning Association.

B

- Lower your body until your chest nearly touches the floor.
- Pause at the bottom, and then push yourself back to the starting position as quickly as possible.
- If your hips sag at any point during the exercise, your form has broken down. When this happens, consider that your last repetition and end the set.

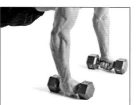

SPARE YOUR WRISTS
If it hurts your wrists to put your hands directly on the floor, place a pair of hex dumbbells at the spots where you position your hands. Then grasp the dumbbells' handles and keep your wrists straight as you perform the exercise.

MUSCLE MISTAKE
You Overwork Your Pecs

Or perhaps more accurately, you work your chest significantly harder than the muscles of your upper back. This can lead to muscle and joint imbalances that result in poor posture and an increased risk of injury. A good rule of thumb: Do a similar number of sets for your upper back as you do for your chest. And if you already have poor posture, devote an even greater proportion of your training time to your upper back muscles.

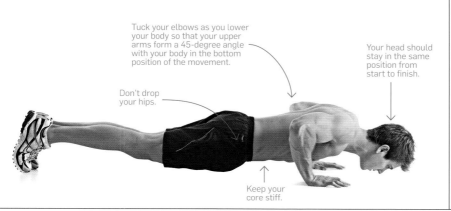

Tuck your elbows as you lower your body so that your upper arms form a 45-degree angle with your body in the bottom position of the movement.

Your head should stay in the same position from start to finish.

Don't drop your hips.

Keep your core stiff.

5

Chest | PUSHUPS

VARIATION #1
Incline Pushup
- Place your hands on a box, bench, or step instead of the floor. This reduces the amount of your body weight you have to lift, making the exercise easier.

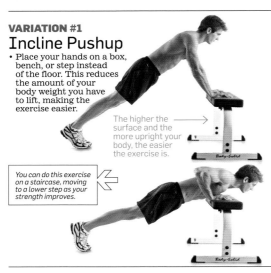

The higher the surface and the more upright your body, the easier the exercise is.

You can do this exercise on a staircase, moving to a lower step as your strength improves.

VARIATION #2
Modified Pushup
- Instead of performing the exercise with your legs straight, bend your knees and cross your ankles behind you. This is another way to make the classic pushup easier.

65
Percent of your body weight you lift when you do a modified pushup.

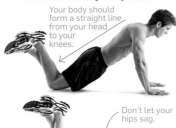

Your body should form a straight line from your head to your knees.

Don't let your hips sag.

VARIATION #3
Decline Pushup
- Place your feet on a box or bench as you perform a pushup. This increases the amount of your body weight you have to lift, making the exercise harder.

STRENGTHEN YOUR SHOULDERS
Researchers in Texas found that the decline pushup works the muscles that stabilize your shoulders better than a traditional pushup.

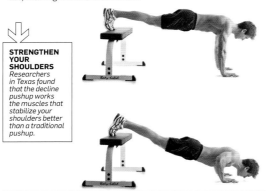

VARIATION #4
Single-Leg Decline Pushup
- Place one foot on a box or bench and hold the other in the air.

PUSH AWAY FAT
The pushup is a good indicator of whether or not you're exercising enough now to avoid fat later, according to a Canadian study. The researchers found that people who perform poorly in a pushup test are 78 percent more likely to gain 20 pounds of flab over the next 2 decades.

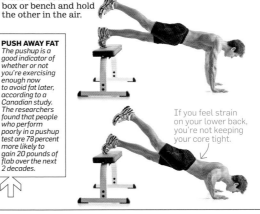

If you feel strain on your lower back, you're not keeping your core tight.

VARIATION #5
Pushup with Feet on Swiss Ball

A

- Perform the movement with your feet placed on a Swiss ball.

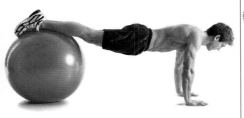

B

- Lower your body as far as you can, without allowing your hips to sag.

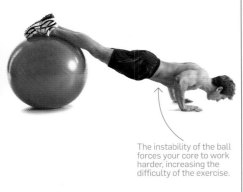

The instability of the ball forces your core to work harder, increasing the difficulty of the exercise.

VARIATION #6
Stacked-Feet Pushup
- Place one foot on top of the other so that only the lower one supports your body.

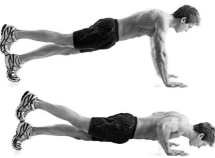

VARIATION #7
Weighted Pushup
- Have a workout partner place a weight plate on your back, at the level of your shoulder blades.

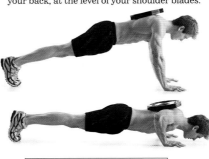

You can also increase the amount you're lifting by wearing a weighted vest or placing a heavy chain on your back.

The Pushup Spectrum

HARDEST

- 9. SWISS-BALL PUSHUP
- 8. BOSU PUSHUP
- 7. SINGLE-LEG DECLINE PUSHUP
- 6. PUSHUP WITH FEET ON SWISS BALL
- 5. DECLINE PUSHUP
- 4. STACKED-FEET PUSHUP
- 3. PUSHUP
- 2. INCLINE PUSHUP
- 1. MODIFIED PUSHUP

EASIEST

Chest | PUSHUPS

VARIATION #8
Triple-Stop Pushup

A

- Do a standard pushup, but pause for 2 seconds at the positions shown.

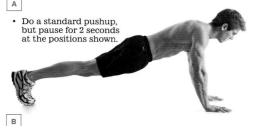

B

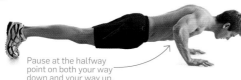

Pause at the halfway point on both your way down and your way up.

C

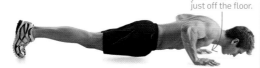

Pause when your chest is just off the floor.

D

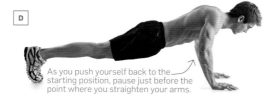

As you push yourself back to the starting position, pause just before the point where you straighten your arms.

MAKE TIME FOR THIS MOVE
Pausing briefly at each point increases strength at that joint angle and 10 degrees in either direction. So this method eliminates any weak point you might have. It also increases the time your muscles are under tension, stimulating growth.

VARIATION #9
Wide-Hands Pushup
- Place your hands about twice shoulder-width apart.

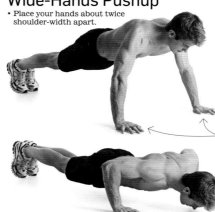

Setting your hands wide puts a greater emphasis on your chest. The downside: It also increases the stress on your shoulders.

VARIATION #10
Close-Hands Pushup
- Place your hands directly under your shoulders.

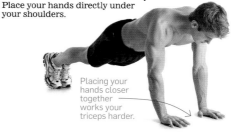

Placing your hands closer together works your triceps harder.

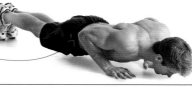

Keep your elbows tucked close to your sides as you lower your body.

VARIATION #11
Diamond Pushup

- Place your hands close enough together to make a triangle with your thumbs and forefingers.

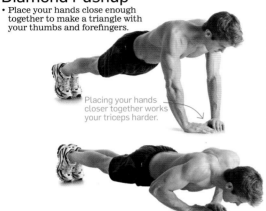

Placing your hands closer together works your triceps harder.

VARIATION #12
Staggered-Hands Pushup

- Place one hand in standard pushup position and your other hand a few inches farther forward.

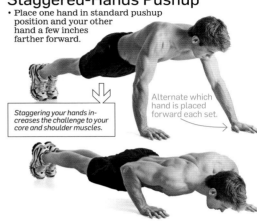

Staggering your hands increases the challenge to your core and shoulder muscles.

Alternate which hand is placed forward each set.

VARIATION #13
Spiderman Pushup

A

- Assume the standard pushup position.

B

- As you lower your body toward the floor, lift your right foot off the floor, swing your right leg out sideways, and try to touch your knee to your elbow.
- Reverse the movement, then push your body back to the starting position. Repeat, but on your next repetition, touch your left knee to your left elbow. Continue to alternate back and forth.

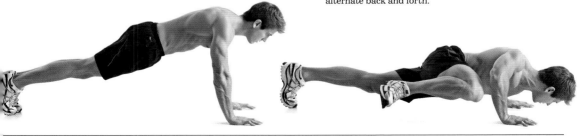

Chest | PUSHUPS

VARIATION #14
Swiss-Ball Pushup
- Place your hands on a Swiss ball instead of the floor.

TARGET YOUR TRICEPS
This exercise trains your triceps 30 percent harder than a standard pushup. The reason: The Swiss ball forces your triceps to stabilize your elbow and shoulder joints, which results in the recruitment of more muscle fibers.

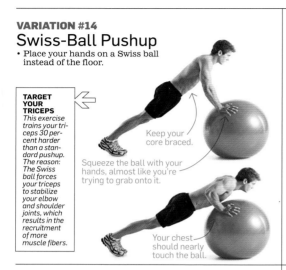

Keep your core braced.

Squeeze the ball with your hands, almost like you're trying to grab onto it.

Your chest should nearly touch the ball.

VARIATION #15
Medicine-Ball Pushup
- Place both hands on a medicine ball.

CHISEL YOUR ABS
When you place your hands on a Swiss ball or a medicine ball, the instability causes your core muscles to work 20 percent harder than when you do pushups on the floor, report New Zealand researchers.

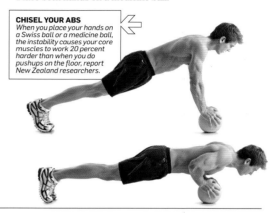

VARIATION #16
Single-Arm Medicine-Ball Pushup
- Place one hand on a medicine ball.

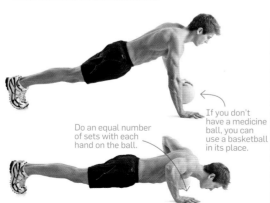

Do an equal number of sets with each hand on the ball.

If you don't have a medicine ball, you can use a basketball in its place.

VARIATION #17
Two-Arm Medicine-Ball Pushup
- Place each hand on a medicine ball.

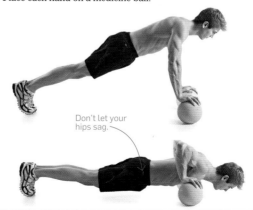

Don't let your hips sag.

VARIATION #18
T-Pushup

A

- Place a pair of hex dumbbells at the spot where you position your hands.
- Grasp the dumbbell handles and set yourself in pushup position.

Set your feet hip-width apart.

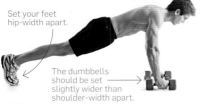

The dumbbells should be set slightly wider than shoulder-width apart.

B

- Lower your body to the floor.

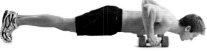

C

- As you push yourself back up, rotate the right side of your body upward as you bend your right arm and pull the right dumbbell to your torso. Then straighten your arm so that the dumbbell is above your right shoulder.

Raise the dumbbell and rotate your body in one fluid motion.

- Lower the dumbbell back down, and repeat, this time performing the move to your left.

As you rotate your body, pivot on your toes and then lower your heels to the floor.

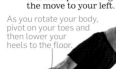

Your arms should form a T with your body.

VARIATION #19
Judo Pushup

A

- Begin in standard pushup position, but move your feet forward and raise your hips so your body almost forms an upside-down V.

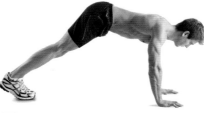

B

- Keeping your hips elevated, lower your body until your chin nearly touches the floor.

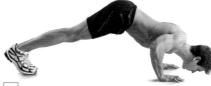

C

- Lower your hips until they almost touch the floor, as you simultaneously raise your head and shoulders toward the ceiling. Reverse the movement back to the starting position and repeat.

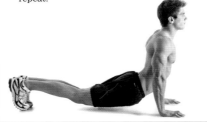

Pump Up Your Pushups

To boost the number of pushups you can do, try this simple ladder routine. Time how long it takes you to do as many push-ups (you can use any varia-tion) as you can. Then rest for the same time period, and repeat the process two to four times. So if you do 20 push-ups in 25 sec-onds, you'll rest 25 seconds, and repeat. Let's say on your next round you complete 12 pushups in 16 seconds. You'd then rest for 16 seconds before your third set. Use this method 2 days a week to quickly raise your score.

11

Chest | PUSHUPS

VARIATION #20
Explosive Pushup

A

- Assume a pushup position.

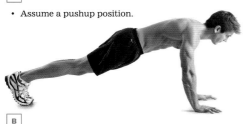

B

- Bend your elbows and lower your body.

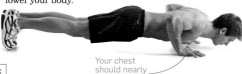

Your chest should nearly touch the floor.

C

- Press yourself up so forcefully that your hands leave the floor.

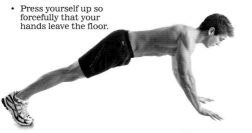

VARIATION #21
Iso-Explosive Pushup

- Do this movement just like the explosive pushup, but first pause for 5 seconds in the down position. This pause technique eliminates all the elasticity in your muscles, which allows you to activate a maximum number of fast-twitch muscle fibers. These are the muscle fibers with the greatest potential for size and strength gains.

VARIATION #22
Explosive Crossover Pushup

A

- Place your left hand on the floor and your right hand on the smooth side of a weight plate.

B

- Lower your body to the floor.

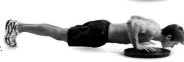

C

- Explosively push up and to the right so your hands leave the floor.

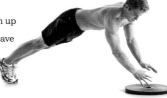

D

- Land with your left hand on the plate and your right hand on the floor.

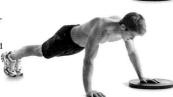

E

- Then lower and repeat, alternating back and forth each repetition.

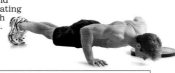

The crossover portion of this movement forces your upper arms toward the center of your body, which is the main function of the pectoralis major, your largest chest muscle.

VARIATION #23
Bosu Pushup

- Turn a Bosu ball over, so that the half-ball portion is on the floor, and position your hands on the sides of the platform.

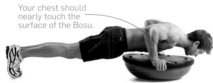

Brace your core and glutes.

Your chest should nearly touch the surface of the Bosu.

VARIATION #24
Suspended Pushup

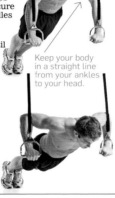

- Attach a pair of straps with handles to a secure bar, so that the handles are a foot or so off the floor.
- Lower your body until your upper arms dip below your elbows.

Keep your body in a straight line from your ankles to your head.

One option for suspended pushups: Blast Straps, which can be found at elitefts.com

Hang On for More Muscle

Performing pushups while suspended from straps increases muscle activation in your abs and upper back, according to a study by Canadian researchers. One caution: This exercise can also place more stress on your lower back. To protect your spine, make sure to keep your core and glutes tight, as you should when you do any variation of the pushup. Simply brace your abs forcefully and squeeze your glutes, and hold those contractions as you lower and raise your body.

VARIATION #25
Pushup and Row

A

- Place a pair of hex dumbbells at the spot where you position your hands.
- Grasp the dumbbell handles and set yourself in pushup position.

B

- Lower your body to the floor, pause, then push yourself back up.

C

- Once you're back in the starting position, row the dumbbell in your right hand to the side of your chest by pulling it upward and bending your arm.
- Pause, then lower the dumbbell back down, and repeat the same movement with your left arm. That's one repetition.

The dumbbells should be set slightly wider than shoulder-width apart.

THE ALL-IN-ONE UPPER BODY EXERCISE
The pushup and row works your middle and upper back as hard as it does your chest.

Your torso should not rotate as you row.

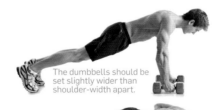
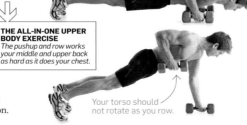

PRESSES

These exercises target your pectoralis major, the largest muscle of your chest. Most of the movements also hit your front deltoids and triceps, since these muscles assist in just about every version of the exercise. Your rotator cuff and trapezius also contract to help keep your shoulders stable as you perform the moves.

TRAINER'S TIP
Imagine that you're pushing your body away from the bar, instead of pushing the bar away from your body. This simple mind trick automatically encourages your body to use good form.

MAIN MOVE
Barbell Bench Press

A

- Grasp a barbell with an overhand grip that's just wider than shoulder-width, and hold it above your sternum with arms completely straight.

As you push the bar off your chest, squeeze and press the bar outward, as if you were trying to tear it apart. This forces more muscle fibers into play.

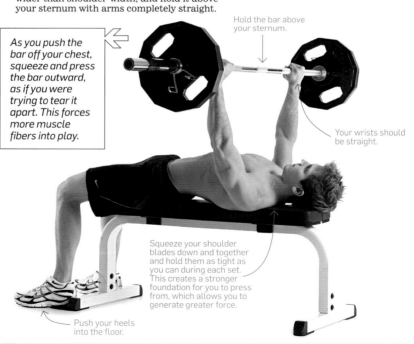

Hold the bar above your sternum.

Your wrists should be straight.

Squeeze your shoulder blades down and together and hold them as tight as you can during each set. This creates a stronger foundation for you to press from, which allows you to generate greater force.

Push your heels into the floor.

WHY FORM MATTERS

Pay closer attention to your exercise technique and you may notice something: People who review proper lifting form before bench-pressing may increase barbell velocity by 183 percent, report researchers at Barry University. The benefit: Faster bar speed helps you blast through sticking points, allowing you to lift heavier loads.

B

- Lower the bar straight down, pause, then press the bar in a straight line back up to the starting position.

- Keep your elbows tucked in, so that your upper arms form a 45-degree angle with your body in the down position. This reduces stress on your shoulder joints.

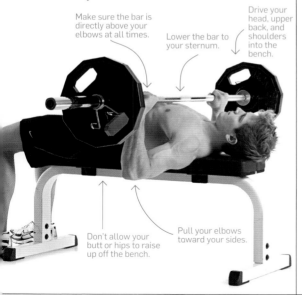

Make sure the bar is directly above your elbows at all times.

Lower the bar to your sternum.

Drive your head, upper back, and shoulders into the bench.

Don't allow your butt or hips to raise up off the bench.

Pull your elbows toward your sides.

VARIATION
Close-Grip Barbell Bench Press
• Use an overhand grip that's shoulder-width apart.

MORE TRICEPS!
Using a close grip forces your triceps to work harder. In fact, the close-grip bench press is one of the best exercises for building size and strength in your triceps.

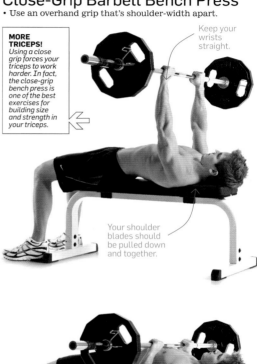

Keep your wrists straight.

Your shoulder blades should be pulled down and together.

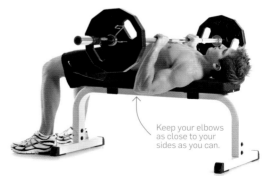

Keep your elbows as close to your sides as you can.

15

Chest | PRESSES

Incline Barbell Bench Press

A

- Set an adjustable bench to its lowest incline, about 15 to 30 degrees.
- Lie faceup on the bench and grab the barbell with an overhand grip that's slightly beyond shoulder width.

Hold the bar above your shoulders.

Your arms should be completely straight.

B

- Lower the bar to your upper chest.
- Pause, and then push the bar back to the starting position.

Keep your wrists straight.

Your feet should be flat on the floor.

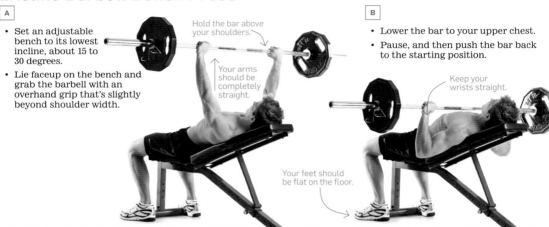

Decline Barbell Bench Press

A

- Lie faceup on a decline bench and grab the barbell with an overhand grip that's slightly beyond shoulder width.
- Hold the bar above your chest with your arms straight.

Your palms should face forward.

B

- Lower the bar to your lower chest.
- Pause, and then push the bar back to the starting position.

The bar should nearly touch your lower chest.

Secure your legs under the anchors.

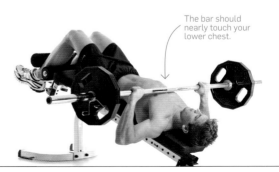

Barbell Floor Press

A

- Lie on the floor instead of on a bench and hold a barbell with an overhand grip.

Your knees should be bent.

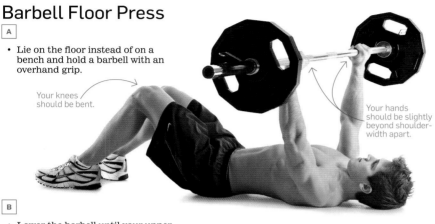

Your hands should be slightly beyond shoulder-width apart.

B

- Lower the barbell until your upper arms touch the floor.
- Keep your elbows pulled in toward your sides as you lower the bar.
- Pause, then push the bar back to the starting position.

Your upper arms should form a 45-degree angle with the sides of your torso.

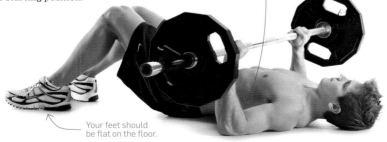

Your feet should be flat on the floor.

MORE ON THE FLOOR!
The floor keeps your upper arms from descending below parallel, which limits your range of motion and concentrates the work on the muscles used during the last (and toughest) part of the bench press.

The Secret of Your Soreness

All of the chest exercises in this chapter work your entire pectoralis major. But you'll notice that when you perform an incline bench press, the upper portion of your chest is the area that's the most sore the next day. For decline bench presses, it's the lower portion. That's because changing the angle of your body puts more tension on a specific segment of your pecs. This causes a greater amount of muscle damage to those fibers, resulting in greater soreness.

Chest | PRESSES

MAIN MOVE
Dumbbell Bench Press

A

- Grab a pair of dumbbells and lie on your back on a flat bench, holding the dumbbells over your chest so that they're nearly touching.

- Your palms should be facing out, but turned slightly inward.

- Before you begin, pull your shoulder blades down and together, and hold them as tight as you can throughout the entire exercise.

B

- Without changing the angle of your hands, lower the dumbbells to the sides of your chest.

- Pause, then press the weights back up to the starting position as quickly as you can.

- Straighten your arms completely at the top of each repetition.

LIFT MORE—TODAY!
UK researchers found that people bench-press 12 percent more weight when they psych themselves up before a lift than when they're distracted. In the study, the scientists gave experienced weight lifters 20 seconds to mentally prepare. The take-home message: Before you approach the bench, skip the small talk and focus on the task at hand.

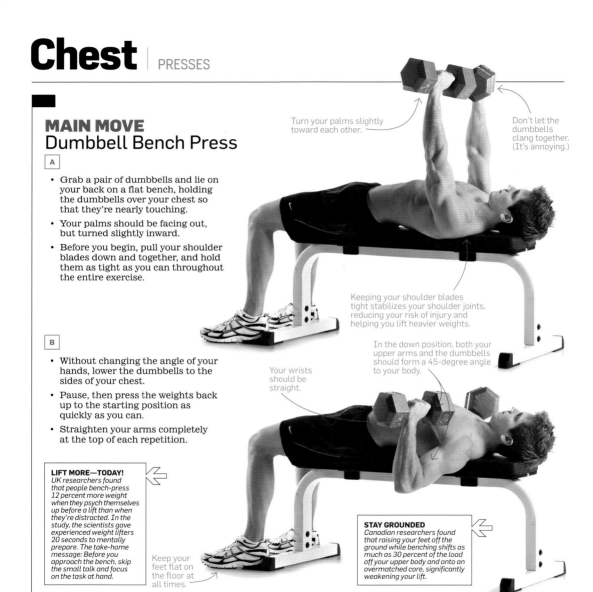

Turn your palms slightly toward each other.

Don't let the dumbbells clang together. (It's annoying.)

Keeping your shoulder blades tight stabilizes your shoulder joints, reducing your risk of injury and helping you lift heavier weights.

In the down position, both your upper arms and the dumbbells should form a 45-degree angle to your body.

Your wrists should be straight.

STAY GROUNDED
Canadian researchers found that raising your feet off the ground while benching shifts as much as 30 percent of the load off your upper body and onto an overmatched core, significantly weakening your lift.

Keep your feet flat on the floor at all times.

VARIATION #1
Alternating Dumbbell Bench Press

- Instead of pressing both dumbbells up at once, lift them one at a time, in an alternating fashion.

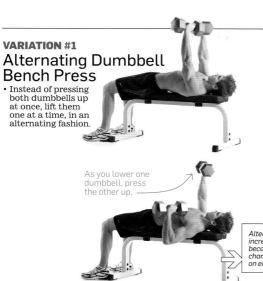

As you lower one dumbbell, press the other up.

Alternating dumbbell presses increase your core activation because you're continually changing the weight distribution on each side of your body.

VARIATION #2
Alternating Neutral-Grip Dumbbell Bench Press

The dumbbells should almost touch.

- Instead of pressing both dumbbells up at once, lift them one at a time, in an alternating fashion. So as you lower one dumbbell, press the other one up.

Your palms should face each other.

VARIATION #3
Neutral-Grip Dumbbell Bench Press

- Hold the dumbbells so that your palms face each other.

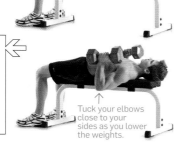

HIT YOUR CHEST HIGHER
Like the incline press, the neutral-grip bench press puts more of the emphasis on your upper chest. So if you don't have an adjustable bench, it's an effective way to target that part of your pectoralis major.

Tuck your elbows close to your sides as you lower the weights.

VARIATION #4
Single-Arm Dumbbell Bench Press

Place your free hand on your abs.

- For this exercise, simply use the same form as for a dumbbell chest press but complete the prescribed number of repetitions with one arm before immediately doing the same number with your other arm.

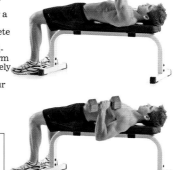

BENCH FOR ABS
Doing any exercise with one dumbbell at a time forces your core to work harder.

19

Chest | PRESSES

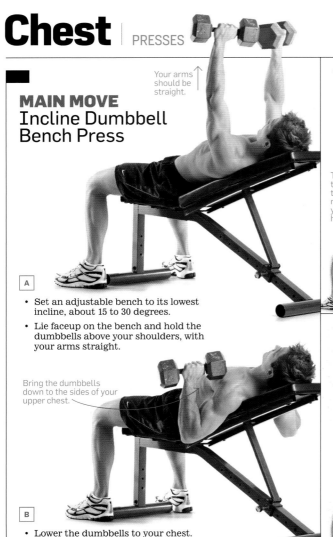

MAIN MOVE
Incline Dumbbell Bench Press

Your arms should be straight. ↑

A

- Set an adjustable bench to its lowest incline, about 15 to 30 degrees.
- Lie faceup on the bench and hold the dumbbells above your shoulders, with your arms straight.

Bring the dumbbells down to the sides of your upper chest.

B

- Lower the dumbbells to your chest.
- Pause, then press the weights back up to the starting position.

VARIATION #1
Neutral-Grip Incline Dumbbell Bench Press
- Hold the dumbbells so that your palms face each other.

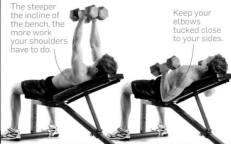

The steeper the incline of the bench, the more work your shoulders have to do.

Keep your elbows tucked close to your sides.

VARIATION #2
Alternating Incline Dumbbell Bench Press
- Instead of pressing both dumbbells up at once, lift them one at a time, in an alternating fashion.

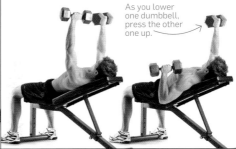

As you lower one dumbbell, press the other one up.

Decline Dumbbell Bench Press

- Grab a pair of dumbbells and lie faceup on a decline bench.
- Hold the dumbbells above your chest.

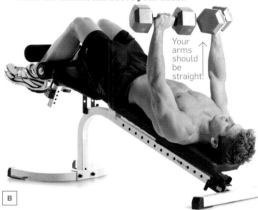

Your arms should be straight.

- Lower the dumbbells to the sides of your lower chest.
- Pause, then press the weights back up to the starting position.

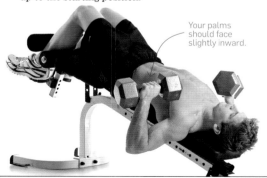

Your palms should face slightly inward.

Dumbbell Floor Press

- Grab a pair of dumbbells and lie faceup on the floor.
- Hold the dumbbells above your chest with your arms straight.

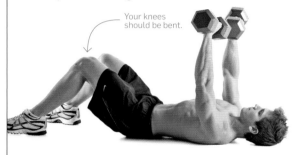

Your knees should be bent.

- Lower the dumbbells until your upper arms touch the floor.
- Pause, then press the weights back up to the starting position.

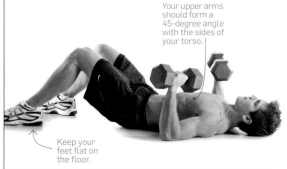

Your upper arms should form a 45-degree angle with the sides of your torso.

Keep your feet flat on the floor.

Chest | FLYS

These exercises target your pectoralis major. Your front deltoids assist in the movements.

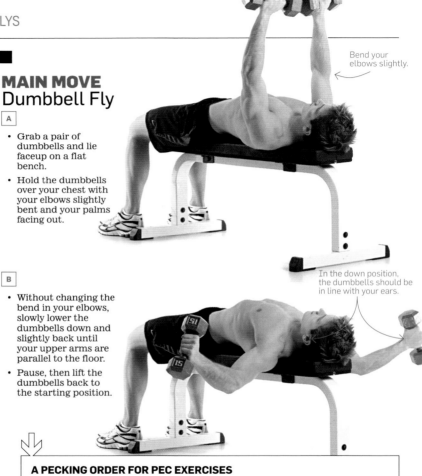

MAIN MOVE
Dumbbell Fly

A

- Grab a pair of dumbbells and lie faceup on a flat bench.
- Hold the dumbbells over your chest with your elbows slightly bent and your palms facing out.

Bend your elbows slightly.

B

- Without changing the bend in your elbows, slowly lower the dumbbells down and slightly back until your upper arms are parallel to the floor.
- Pause, then lift the dumbbells back to the starting position.

In the down position, the dumbbells should be in line with your ears.

A PECKING ORDER FOR PEC EXERCISES
The chest fly is best placed at the end of your workout. Researchers at Truman State University found that pectoral muscles are activated for 23 percent less time during the chest fly than during the bench press. As a result, the scientists say that dumbbell and barbell chest presses can be used interchangeably but that the fly shouldn't be your primary lift for working your chest.

VARIATION #1
Incline Dumbbell Fly
• Lie faceup on a bench set to a low incline.

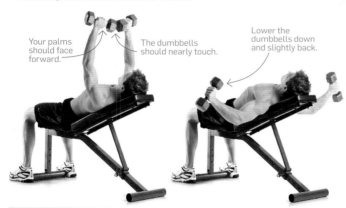

Your palms should face forward.

The dumbbells should nearly touch.

Lower the dumbbells down and slightly back.

VARIATION #2
Incline Dumbbell Fly to Press
• This exercise combines the incline fly with an incline press. Start by doing the incline fly, performing as many repetitions as you can until you start to struggle. Then immediately switch to incline dumbbell presses and complete as many repetitions as you can with perfect form.

MUSCLE MISTAKE
You Still Use the Chest Fly Machine

The chest fly machine, also known as the pec deck, can overstretch the front of your shoulder and cause the muscles around the rear of your shoulder to stiffen. The result is a higher risk for a painful injury called shoulder impingement syndrome. So skip the fly machine, and stick with the exercises in this chapter instead. For any exercise, perform it only if you can complete it pain-free for the full range of motion.

VARIATION #3
Decline Dumbbell Fly
• Lie faceup on a decline bench.

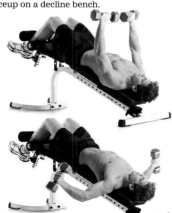

VARIATION #4
Swiss-Ball Dumbbell Fly
• Lie with your middle and upper back placed firmly on a Swiss ball.

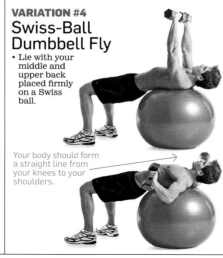

Your body should form a straight line from your knees to your shoulders.

Chest

THE BEST CHEST EXERCISE YOU'VE NEVER DONE
Pushup Plus

Besides working your chest, this exercise is highly effective at engaging your serratus anterior, a small but important muscle that helps move your shoulder blades. Neglect this muscle, as most guys do, and it becomes weak. That puts you at high risk for shoulder impingement— a painful injury in which a muscle tendon becomes entrapped in your shoulder joint. What's more, serratus anterior weakness often causes your shoulder blades to tilt forward and down, resulting in rounded shoulders— giving you a permanent slump.

Now, the classic pushup does work your serratus anterior. But adding the "plus"— pushing your upper back toward the ceiling at the end of the movement— makes the exercise even more effective. In fact, University of Minnesota researchers found that the pushup plus activates your serratus anterior 38 percent more than the standard pushup does.

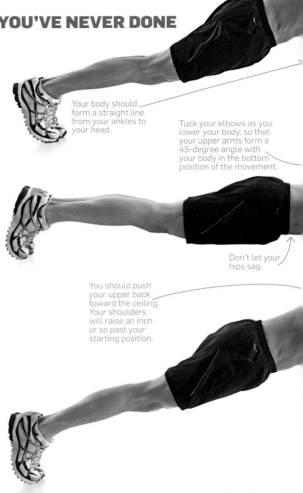

Your body should form a straight line from your ankles to your head.

Tuck your elbows as you lower your body, so that your upper arms form a 45-degree angle with your body in the bottom position of the movement.

Don't let your hips sag.

You should push your upper back toward the ceiling. Your shoulders will raise an inch or so past your starting position.

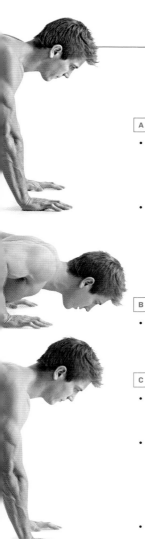

A

- Get down on all fours and place your hands on the floor so that they're slightly wider than and in line with your shoulders.
- Brace your abdominals—as if you were about to be punched in the gut—and hold them that way for the duration of this exercise.

B

- Lower your body until your chest nearly touches the floor.

C

- Pause, and then push yourself back to the starting position as quickly as possible.
- Once your arms are straight again, push your upper back toward the ceiling. The movement is very slight; it's hard to see, but you'll feel the difference.
- Pause for a count of one, then do another pushup and repeat.

BONUS EXERCISE!
Swiss-Ball Pushup Plus

A

- Place your hands directly under your shoulders and on the sides of a Swiss ball.

B

- Keeping your core tight, lower yourself until your chest grazes the ball, then push back up.

C

- Perform the "plus" by pushing your upper back away from the ball.

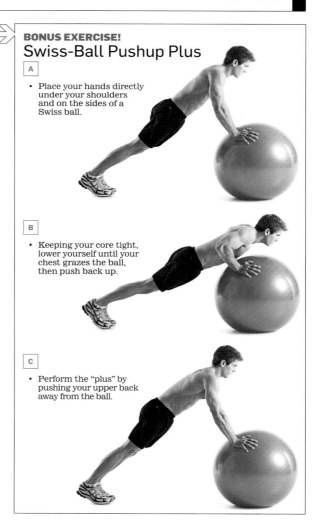

Back

R arely do you hear someone say, "Wow! That guy has a great back!" After all, most men don't spend nearly as much time working their back muscles as they do the muscles on the fronts of their bodies. So even if a guy has a well-developed chest, it's quite likely that he's neglecting his back, by comparison. And that leads to a problem: poor posture. When your chest muscles are stronger than your back muscles, the resulting imbalance pulls your shoulders forward, leaving you with a hunched back.

The good news: By focusing more on your back, you can straighten your posture and look as fit when you're walking away as you do on your approach.

Bonus Benefits

A bigger bench press! The muscles of your upper- and mid-back are key for stabilizing your shoulder joints. And strong, stable shoulders allow you to lift heavier weights in just about every upper-body exercise, from the bench press to the arm curl.

Bulging biceps! Exercises that work your back are also great for targeting your arms. That's because any time that you have to bend your elbows to lift a weight, you're training your biceps—whether you're doing an arm curl or a classic "back" exercise such as a row or chinup. Think about it: How would your *arms* know the difference?

A leaner midsection! Building your back can torch belly fat. It's metabolism 101: The more muscles you train, the more calories you burn.

Meet Your Muscles

Rear Deltoid

While your rear deltoid [1] is typically thought of as a shoulder muscle (and you'll learn more about it in Chapter 3), it's actually emphasized by many of the exercises that work your upper back. That's because its job is to pull your upper arm backward, a movement that you perform whenever you do a rowing exercise.

Teres Major

The teres major [2] starts on the outer edge of your shoulder blade, or scapula, and—like your lats—attaches to the inside of your upper arm. So it assists your lats in pulling your upper arm down to the side of your torso.

Latissimus Dorsi

Your latissimus dorsi [3] originates on the lower half of your back, along your spine and hip, and attaches to the inside of your upper arm. The primary job of your two lats is to pull your upper arms from a raised position down to the sides of your torso, as when you grab an object off a high shelf. That's why exercises that require this movement, such as chinups, pullups, lat pulldowns, and pullovers, are such popular back builders.

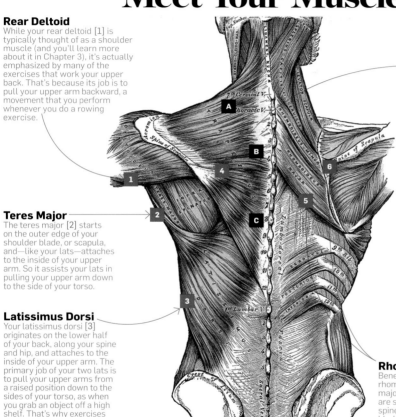

Trapezius

Your trapezius [4] is a long, triangle-shaped muscle located on the upper half of your back. Because of the way its muscle fibers are arranged, it has several jobs.

The upper portion of your traps [A] are responsible for lifting your shoulder blades. This allows you to shrug your shoulders. It's worth noting that the best movements for working these fibers—lateral raises and shrugs—are classified as shoulder exercises and are found in Chapter 3.

The middle portion of your traps [B], with fibers running perpendicular to your spine, are responsible for pulling your shoulder blades closer together, toward the middle of your back. Rowing exercises emphasize these muscle fibers.

The lower portion of your traps [C], with fibers ascending to your shoulder blades, pull your shoulder blades down. Rowing movements work these fibers as well.

Rhomboids

Beneath your trapezius lie your rhomboids, specifically the rhomboid major [5] and rhomboid minor. [6] These are small muscles that start at your spine and attach to your shoulder blades. They assist your traps with pulling your shoulder blades together.

Upper Back | ROWS & RAISES

In this chapter, you'll find 69 exercises that target the muscles of your back. These exercises are divided into two major sections: Upper-Back Exercises and Lat Exercises. Within each section, you'll notice that certain exercises have been given the designation Main Move. Master this basic version of a movement, and you'll be able to do all of its variations with flawless form.

ROWS & RAISES

These exercises target your middle and lower traps, your rhomboid major, and your rhomboid minor. They also hit your upper traps, rear deltoids, and rotator cuff muscles, which assist in the rowing movement or act as stabilizers in every version of these exercises.

MAIN MOVE
Inverted Row

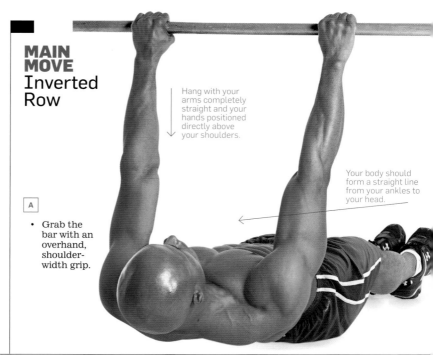

Hang with your arms completely straight and your hands positioned directly above your shoulders.

Your body should form a straight line from your ankles to your head.

A

- Grab the bar with an overhand, shoulder-width grip.

Why Rows Matter

Rowing exercises train your trapezius and rhomboids, muscles that help keep your shoulder blades from moving as you lift a weight. That's important because unstable shoulders can limit your strength in exercises for your chest and arms. For instance, your chest muscles might be capable of bench-pressing 225 pounds, but if your shoulders can't support that weight, you won't be able to complete one rep. So boost your strength on rows to boost your strength all over.

THE REVERSE PUSHUP?

The inverted row is to your back as the pushup is to your chest. Not only is it great for working the muscles of your middle and upper back but it also challenges your core.

If your wrists start to "curl" as you perform the movement—that is, if you have trouble keeping them straight—it's a sign that your upper back and/or your biceps are weak.

Try to keep your wrists straight.

Keep your body rigid for the entire movement.

B

- Initiate the movement by pulling your shoulder blades back, then continue the pull with your arms to lift your chest to the bar.
- Pause, then slowly lower your body back to the starting position.

29

Upper Back

Y-T-L-W-I RAISE
This is a fantastic, multi-part exercise that targets the muscles of your upper back that stabilize your shoulder blades—particularly your trapezius. It also strengthens your shoulder muscles in every direction, emphasizing your rotator cuff and deltoids.

You can perform all parts of the Y-T-L-W-I raise as a *complete* upper-back workout, with or without the dumbbells (depending on your ability). If you don't use weights, make sure your hands are positioned just as if you were holding the dumbbells. When using weights, you'll likely find that all you'll need is, at most, a very light pair of dumbbells. You can do the exercise while lying chest down on an incline bench or a Swiss ball. The ball makes the movements even harder, since it engages your core muscles to help you maintain your position. Three of the movements—Y-T-I—can also be effectively performed on the floor, which can come in handy in a hotel room.

Incline Y Raise

 A

- Set an adjustable bench to a low incline and lie with your chest against the pad.

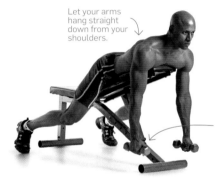

Let your arms hang straight down from your shoulders.

Turn your arms so that your palms are facing each other.

 B

- Raise your arms at a 30-degree angle to your body (so that they form a Y) until they're in line with your body.
- Pause, then slowly lower back to the starting position.

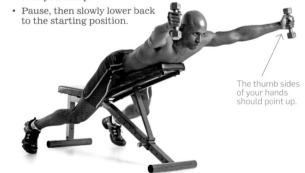

The thumb sides of your hands should point up.

Floor Y Raise

A

- Lie facedown on the floor. Allow your arms to rest on the floor, completely straight and at a 30-degree angle to your body, your palms facing each other.

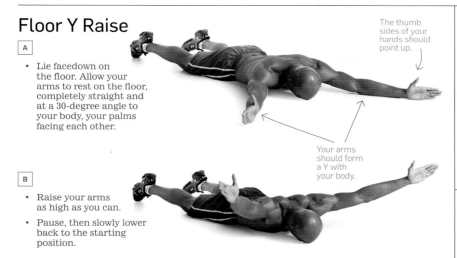

The thumb sides of your hands should point up.

Your arms should form a Y with your body.

B

- Raise your arms as high as you can.

- Pause, then slowly lower back to the starting position.

Swiss-Ball Y Raise

A

- Lie facedown on top of a Swiss ball so that your back is flat and your chest is off the ball.

B

- Raise your arms at a 30-degree angle to your body (so that they form a Y) until they're in line with your body.

- Pause, then slowly lower back to the starting position.

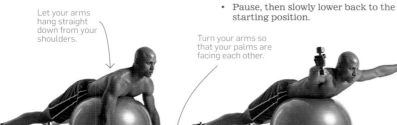

Let your arms hang straight down from your shoulders.

Turn your arms so that your palms are facing each other.

The Complete Upper-Back Workout

Do 10 reps of the Y raise, then immediately do 10 reps of the T raise. Continue on until you've done all five movements of the Y-T-L-W-I raise. Rest for 2 minutes and repeat one time.

The No-Equipment Back Workout

Do 12 repetitions each of Y-T-I while lying facedown on the floor, without resting between movements.

Five More Exercises!

Besides performing Y-T-L-W-I raises on an incline bench, a Swiss ball, and the floor, you can do each of the movements in the same bent-over position in which you do barbell and dumbbell rows. Just make sure to keep your lower back naturally arched as you perform the exercises.

31

Upper Back | ROWS & RAISES

Incline T Raise

- Grab a pair of dumbbells and lie chest down on an adjustable bench set to a low incline.

- Raise your arms straight out to your sides until they're in line with your body.

- Pause, then slowly lower back to the starting position.

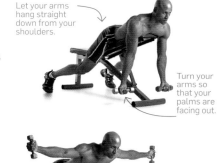

Let your arms hang straight down from your shoulders.

Turn your arms so that your palms are facing out.

The thumb sides of your hands should point up.

Floor T Raise

- Move your arms so that they're out to your sides—perpendicular to your body with the thumb sides of your hands pointing up—and raise them as high as you comfortably can.

- Pause, then slowly lower back to the starting position.

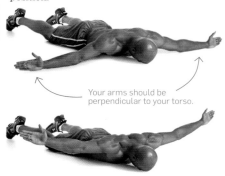

Your arms should be perpendicular to your torso.

Swiss Ball T Raise

A

- Lie facedown on top of a Swiss ball so that your back is flat and your chest is off the ball.

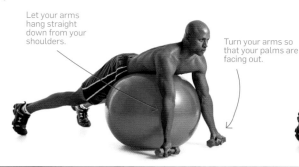

Let your arms hang straight down from your shoulders.

Turn your arms so that your palms are facing out.

B

- Raise your arms straight out to your sides until they're in line with your body.

- Pause, then slowly lower back to the starting position.

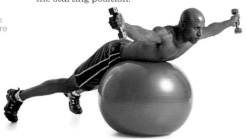

Incline I Raise

- Grab a pair of dumbbells and lie chest down on an adjustable bench set to a low incline.

- Let your arms hang straight down from your shoulders, palms facing each other.

- Raise your arms straight up, so that they're in line with your body and form an I.

- Pause, then slowly lower back to the starting position.

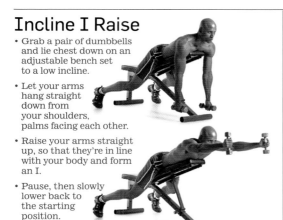

Floor I Raise

- Position your arms straight above your shoulders so your body forms a straight line from your feet to your fingertips.

- Raise your arms as high as you comfortably can.

- Pause, then slowly lower back to the starting position.

Your palms should be facing each other so that the thumb sides of your hands point up.

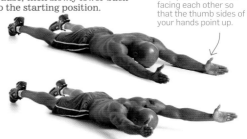

Swiss-Ball I Raise

A

- Grab a pair of dumbbells and lie facedown on top of a Swiss ball so that your back is flat and your chest is off the ball.

B

- Raise your arms straight up, so that they're in line with your body and form an I.

- Pause, then slowly lower back to the starting position.

Turn your arms so that your palms are facing each other.

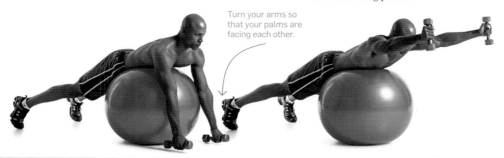

Upper Back | ROWS & RAISES

MAIN MOVE
Barbell Row

A

- Grab the barbell with an overhand grip that's just beyond shoulder width, and hold it at arm's length.

- Bend at your hips and knees and lower your torso until it's almost parallel to the floor.

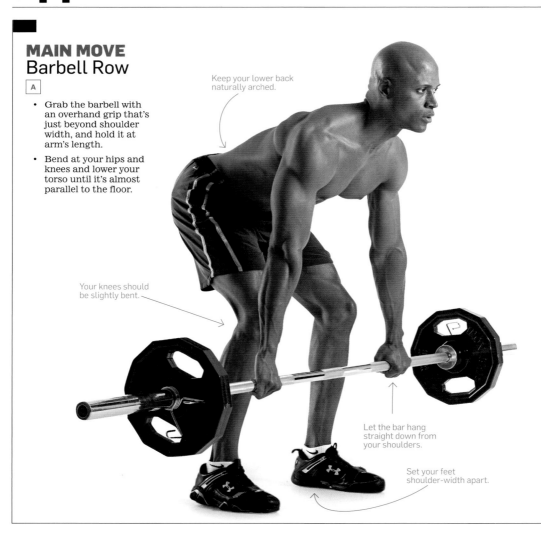

Keep your lower back naturally arched.

Your knees should be slightly bent.

Let the bar hang straight down from your shoulders.

Set your feet shoulder-width apart.

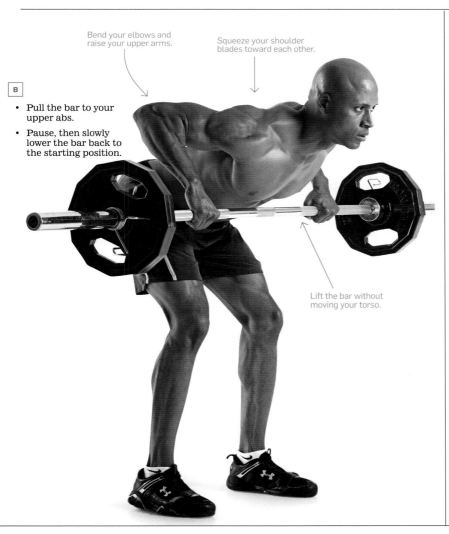

Bend your elbows and raise your upper arms.

Squeeze your shoulder blades toward each other.

B

- Pull the bar to your upper abs.
- Pause, then slowly lower the bar back to the starting position.

Lift the bar without moving your torso.

MUSCLE MISTAKE
You Round Your Lower Back When You Row

This mistake can lead to injuries such as herniated disks. Here's how to avoid it: Pick up the weight and stand tall—with your lower back naturally arched. Keeping your upper body rigid, bend your knees slightly as you push your hips backward as far as possible. Then without changing the posture of your torso, lower your upper body until it's nearly parallel to the floor. Now check your form in the mirror.

Upper Back |

Mix and match one of four grip positions—overhand, neutral, underhand, elbows-out—with any of the eight versions of the dumbbell row that follow. All of the grips are interchangeable with each type of row, giving you 32 back-building options from this one classic move.

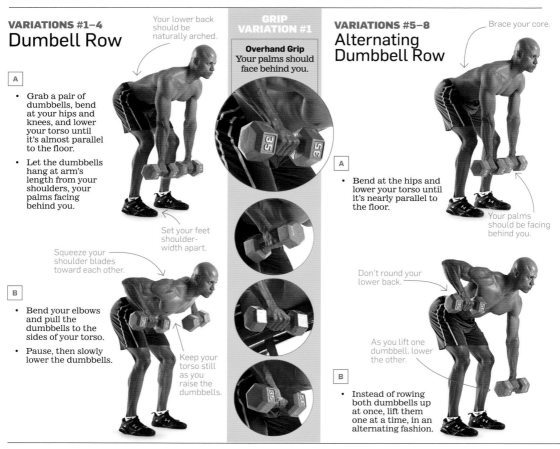

VARIATIONS #1–4
Dumbell Row

Your lower back should be naturally arched.

A

- Grab a pair of dumbbells, bend at your hips and knees, and lower your torso until it's almost parallel to the floor.

- Let the dumbbells hang at arm's length from your shoulders, your palms facing behind you.

Set your feet shoulder-width apart.

Squeeze your shoulder blades toward each other.

B

- Bend your elbows and pull the dumbbells to the sides of your torso.

- Pause, then slowly lower the dumbbells.

Keep your torso still as you raise the dumbbells.

GRIP VARIATION #1

Overhand Grip
Your palms should face behind you.

VARIATIONS #5–8
Alternating Dumbbell Row

Brace your core.

A

- Bend at the hips and lower your torso until it's nearly parallel to the floor.

Your palms should be facing behind you.

Don't round your lower back.

As you lift one dumbbell, lower the other.

B

- Instead of rowing both dumbbells up at once, lift them one at a time, in an alternating fashion.

VARIATIONS #9–12
Single-Leg Neutral-Grip Dumbbell Row

A

- Bend at the hips and lower your torso until it's nearly parallel to the floor.

Your lower back should be naturally arched.

- Raise one leg and hold it in the air.

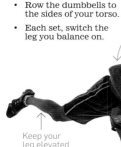

Your palms should be facing each other.

B

- Row the dumbbells to the sides of your torso.
- Each set, switch the leg you balance on.

Tuck your elbows close to your sides.

Keep your leg elevated as you row.

GRIP VARIATION #2

Neutral Grip
Your palms should face each other. When you row the weight, keep your elbows close to your sides.

VARIATIONS #13–16
Single-Arm Neutral-Grip Dumbbell Row

Brace your core.

Place your free hand behind your back, palm facing up.

A

- Grab a dumbbell in your right hand, bend at your hips and knees, and lower your torso until it's almost parallel to the floor.
- Let the dumbbell hang at arm's length from your shoulders.

Use a neutral grip, so that your right palm is facing left.

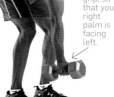

The single-arm row allows you to work each side of your body separately, helping to shore up muscle imbalances while increasing the challenge to your core.

B

- Pull the dumbell to the side of your torso, keeping your elbow tucked close to your side.

Don't rotate or lift your torso as you row the weight.

Bend your knees slightly.

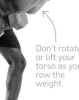

37

Upper Back |

VARIATIONS #17–20
Lying Supported Elbows-Out Dumbbell Row

A

- Instead of standing, perform the exercise while lying chest down on a bench set to its lowest incline.

- Let the dumbbells hang at arm's length from your shoulders.

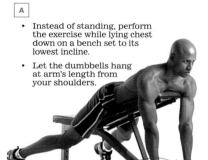

Your palms should be facing behind you.

B

- Keeping your elbows flared out, row the dumbbells toward the sides of your chest.

Keep your lower back naturally arched as you perform the movement, instead of allowing your upper body to "collapse" against the bench.

Your upper arms should be perpendicular to your body.

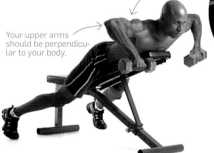

GRIP VARIATION #3

Elbows-Out Overhand Grip
Your palms should face behind you. As you row, keep your elbows flared so your upper arm is perpendicular to your torso.

VARIATIONS #21–24
Kneeling Supported Elbows-Out Single-Arm Dumbbell Row

A

Don't round your lower back.

- Place your left hand and left knee on a flat bench.

- Your lower back should be naturally arched and your torso parallel to the floor.

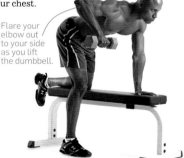

Your palms should be facing behind you.

B

- Keeping your upper arm perpendicular to your body, row the weight toward the side of your chest.

Flare your elbow out to your side as you lift the dumbbell.

VARIATIONS #25–28
Single-Arm, Single-Leg Underhand-Grip Dumbbell Row

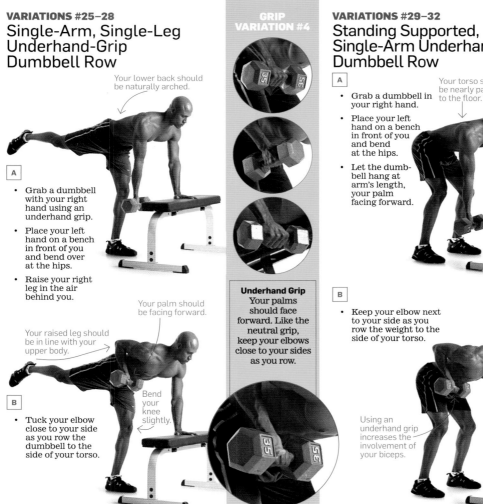

Your lower back should be naturally arched.

A

- Grab a dumbbell with your right hand using an underhand grip.
- Place your left hand on a bench in front of you and bend over at the hips.
- Raise your right leg in the air behind you.

Your raised leg should be in line with your upper body.

Your palm should be facing forward.

Bend your knee slightly.

B

- Tuck your elbow close to your side as you row the dumbbell to the side of your torso.

GRIP VARIATION #4

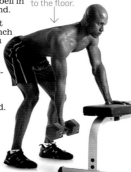

Underhand Grip
Your palms should face forward. Like the neutral grip, keep your elbows close to your sides as you row.

VARIATIONS #29–32
Standing Supported, Single-Arm Underhand-Grip Dumbbell Row

A

- Grab a dumbbell in your right hand.
- Place your left hand on a bench in front of you and bend at the hips.
- Let the dumbbell hang at arm's length, your palm facing forward.

Your torso should be nearly parallel to the floor.

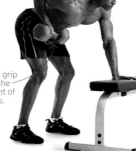

B

- Keep your elbow next to your side as you row the weight to the side of your torso.

Using an underhand grip increases the involvement of your biceps.

Upper Back | ROWS & RAISES

MAIN MOVE
Rear Lateral Raise

A

- Grab a pair of dumbbells and bend forward at your hips until your torso is nearly parallel to the floor.

- Let the dumbbells hang straight down from your shoulders, your palms facing each other.

B

- Without moving your torso, raise your arms straight out to your sides until they're in line with your body.

- Pause, then slowly return to the starting position.

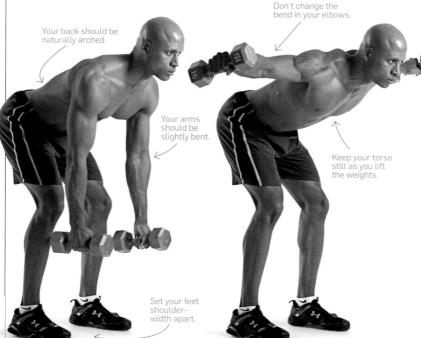

Your back should be naturally arched.

Your arms should be slightly bent.

Set your feet shoulder-width apart.

Don't change the bend in your elbows.

Keep your torso still as you lift the weights.

The Most Surprising Back Exercise?

Most people think of the rear lateral raise as strictly a shoulder exercise, since it targets your rear deltoid. But consider: It's actually the same movement as a row, only you're not bending your elbows as you lift the weight. So it's also highly effective at working the muscles of your middle and upper back, which is why it's included in this chapter. For best results, focus on squeezing your shoulder blades together as you do the exercise.

VARIATION #1
Underhand-Grip Rear Lateral Raise

- Perform the movement with an underhand grip. Your palms should be facing forward, instead of facing each other.

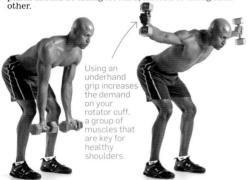

Using an underhand grip increases the demand on your rotator cuff, a group of muscles that are key for healthy shoulders.

VARIATION #2
Overhand-Grip Rear Lateral Raise

- Perform the movement while holding the dumbbells with an overhand grip. Your palms should be facing behind you, instead of facing each other.

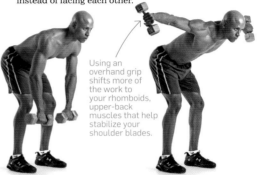

Using an overhand grip shifts more of the work to your rhomboids, upper-back muscles that help stabilize your shoulder blades.

VARIATION #3
Seated Rear Lateral Raise

- Grab a pair of dumbbells and sit at the end of a bench, instead of standing.

Keep your lower back naturally arched.

Raise your arms straight out to your sides.

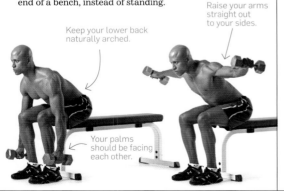

Your palms should be facing each other.

VARIATION #4
Lying Dumbbell Raise

- Grab a dumbbell in your right hand and lie on your left side on a flat bench.
- Prop yourself up with your left elbow.
- Let your right arm hang straight down so that it's perpendicular to the floor, with your palm facing behind you and your elbow slightly bent.
- Without changing the bend in your elbow, raise your arm straight above your shoulder while rotating your arm so that your palm is facing your head.
- Slowly return to the starting position.

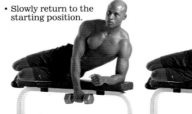

Upper Back | ROWS & RAISES

MAIN MOVE
Cable Row

- Attach a straight bar to the cable and position yourself with your feet braced.
- Grab the bar with an overhand grip that's just beyond shoulder width.

Sit up straight and push your chest out and pull your shoulders down and back.

Your knees should be slightly bent.

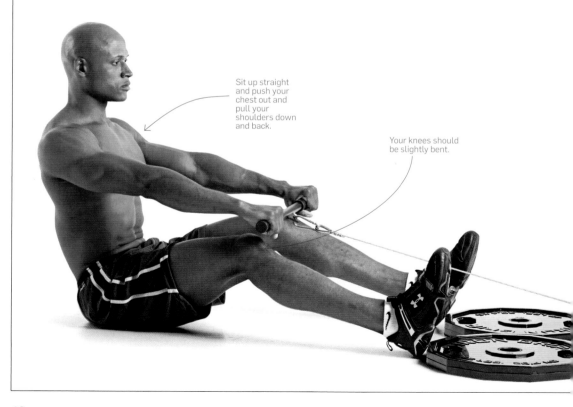

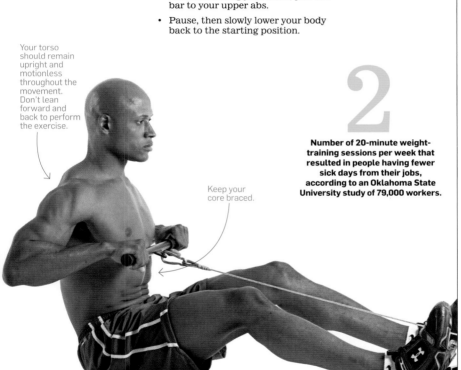

B

- Without moving your torso, pull the bar to your upper abs.

- Pause, then slowly lower your body back to the starting position.

Your torso should remain upright and motionless throughout the movement. Don't lean forward and back to perform the exercise.

Keep your core braced.

2

Number of 20-minute weight-training sessions per week that resulted in people having fewer sick days from their jobs, according to an Oklahoma State University study of 79,000 workers.

MUSCLE MISTAKE
You Row with High Shoulders

When you do any type of row, start the movement by pulling your shoulders back and down. Why? Because otherwise, you'll tend to keep your shoulders elevated, which allows you to hyperextend them as you row your elbows back. This stresses both the front of your shoulder and a rotator cuff muscle called the subscapularis. Over time, this can cause your shoulder joint to become unstable, which often leads to injuries.

Upper Back |

VARIATION #1
Wide-Grip Cable Row
- Position your hands about 1½ times shoulder-width apart, and pull the bar to your lower chest.

The wider grip increases the involvement of your rear deltoids.

VARIATION #2
Underhand-Grip Cable Row
- Grasp the bar with a shoulder-width, underhand grip and pull the bar to your lower abs.

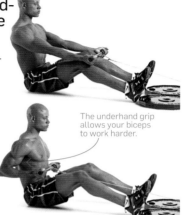

The underhand grip allows your biceps to work harder.

VARIATION #3
Rope-Handle Cable Row
- Attach a rope handle to the cable, grab an end with each hand, and perform a cable row.

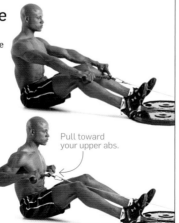

Pull toward your upper abs.

VARIATION #4
V-Grip Cable Row
- Attach a V-grip to the cable, grasp it with both hands, and pull it toward your midsection.

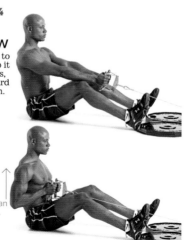

Keep your torso upright; don't lean forward or back.

VARIATION #5
Single-Arm Cable Row

- Attach a stirrup handle to the cable and perform the movement with one arm at a time. Without moving your torso, pull the handle to your side.

- Complete the prescribed number of repetitions to your right side, then immediately do the same number to your left side.

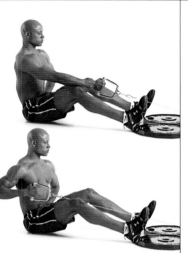

VARIATION #6
Single-Arm Cable Row and Rotation

- Attach a stirrup handle to the cable and grasp it with your right hand.

- Pull the handle toward your right side as you rotate your torso to the right.

- Pause, then reverse the movement back to the starting position.

Sit tall and keep your torso upright.

Keep your core tight as you perform this exercise.

VARIATION #7
Cable Row to Neck with External Rotation

- Attach a rope handle to the cable and position yourself in front of the machine.

- Pull the middle of the rope toward your face as you squeeze your shoulder blades together and rotate your upper arms and forearms up and back.

- Pause, then slowly return to the starting position.

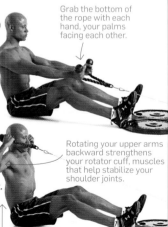

Grab the bottom of the rope with each hand, your palms facing each other.

Rotating your upper arms backward strengthens your rotator cuff, muscles that help stabilize your shoulder joints.

Sit up straight.

VARIATION #8
Standing Single-Arm Cable Row

- Attach a stirrup handle to the low pulley of a cable, grab it with your right hand, and stand in a staggered stance.

- Pull the handle toward your right side as you rotate your torso to the right. Pause, then reverse the movement to the starting position.

- Complete the prescribed number of repetitions to your right side, then immediately do the same number to your left side.

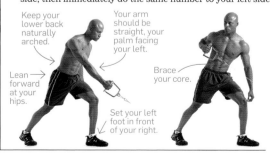

Keep your lower back naturally arched.

Your arm should be straight, your palm facing your left.

Lean forward at your hips.

Brace your core.

Set your left foot in front of your right.

45

CHINUPS & PULLUPS
These exercises target your lats. They also hit your teres major and biceps. What's more, your core and middle and upper back muscles are involved, assisting in the movement or acting as stabilizers in most versions of this exercise.

MAIN MOVE
Chinup

A

- Grab the chinup bar with a shoulder-width, underhand grip.

- Hang at arm's length. You should return to this position—known as a dead hang—each time you lower your body back down.

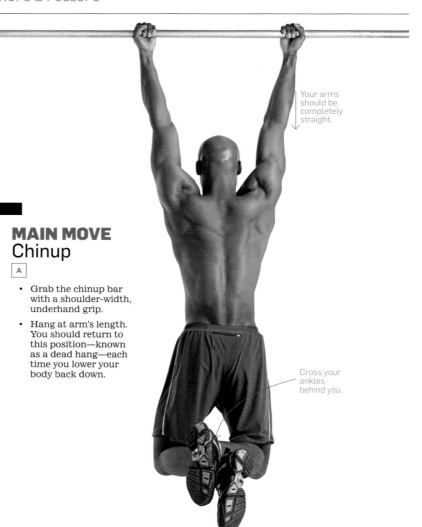

Your arms should be completely straight.

Cross your ankles behind you.

Squeeze your shoulder blades together.

Pull your upper arms down forcefully.

TRAINER'S TIP
Imagine that you're pulling the bar to your chest, instead of your chest to the bar.

 B

- Pull your chest to the bar.
- Once the top of your chest touches the bar, pause, then slowly lower your body back to a dead hang.

MIX YOUR GRIP
Try a mixed grip chinup. Placing your hands shoulder-width apart, use an underhand grip with one hand and an overhand grip with the other.

The Chinup vs the Pullup

In case you're wondering about the difference between a chinup and a pullup, it's simple: For a chinup, you use an underhand grip; for a pullup, you use an overhand grip. Of course, you'll quickly discover that the chinup is a little easier. (Or perhaps "less hard" would be more accurate.) This is because an underhand grip allows your biceps to be more involved with the exercise, providing more total muscle power to pull you up.

Lats |

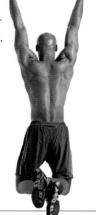

VARIATION #1
Negative Chinup

 A

- Set a bench under a chinup bar, step up on the bench, and grasp the bar using a shoulder-width, underhand grip.

- From the bench, jump up so that your chest is next to your hands, then cross your ankles behind you.

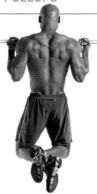

B

- Try to take 5 seconds to lower your body until your arms are straight. If that's too hard, lower yourself as slowly as you can.

- Jump up to the starting position and repeat.

Lower your body at the same rate of speed from the top position of the negative chinup to the bottom. If you notice that you speed up at a specific point, make a mental note. Then, on your next set, pause for a second or two just above that point as you lower your body. This will help you improve your performance faster. A good way to gauge your progress: Once you can complete a 30-second negative chinup, you can probably perform one full standard chinup.

VARIATION #2
Band-Assisted Chinup

A

- Loop one end of a large rubber band around a chinup bar and then pull it through the other end of the band, cinching the band tightly to the bar.

- Grab the bar with a shoulder-width, underhand grip, place your knees in the loop of the band, and hang at arm's length.

B

- Perform a chinup by pulling your chest to the bar.

- Once the top of your chest touches the bar, pause, then slowly lower your body back to a dead hang.

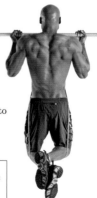

The band-assisted method will allow you to do full chinups, and it more accurately mimics the movement than does the assisted-chinup machine you find in commercial gyms. Try a SuperBand (available at ihpfit.com) or a Jump Stretch Mini Flex Band (which you can find at elitefts.com).

VARIATION #3
Close-Grip Chinup
• Use an underhand grip with your hands placed 6 to 8 inches apart.

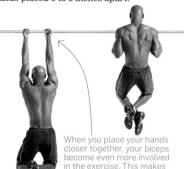

When you place your hands closer together, your biceps become even more involved in the exercise. This makes the exercise easier than the classic chinup.

VARIATION #4
Neutral-Grip Chinup
• Grab the parallel handles of a chinup station, so that your palms are facing each other. Now pull your chest to the level of the bars.

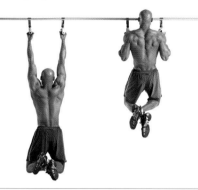

VARIATION #5
Pullup
• This is the same movement as a chinup except that you grab the bar with an overhand grip that's slightly wider than shoulder width.

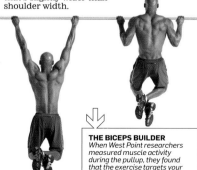

THE BICEPS BUILDER
When West Point researchers measured muscle activity during the pullup, they found that the exercise targets your biceps just as much as your lats.

VARIATION #6
Wide-Grip Pullup
• Use an overhand grip that's about 1½ times shoulder width.

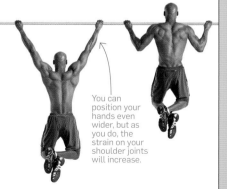

You can position your hands even wider, but as you do, the strain on your shoulder joints will increase.

The Chinup Spectrum

HARDEST

— 8. WIDE-GRIP PULLUP

— 7. PULLUP

— 6. MIXED-GRIP CHINUP

— 5. NEUTRAL-GRIP CHINUP

— 4. CHINUP

— 3. CLOSE-GRIP CHINUP

— 2. BAND-ASSISTED CHINUP

— 1. NEGATIVE CHINUP

EASIEST

49

PULLDOWNS

These exercises target your lats. They also hit your teres major and biceps. What's more, your middle and upper back muscles are involved to varying degrees, assisting in the movement or acting as stabilizers in most versions of the exercises.

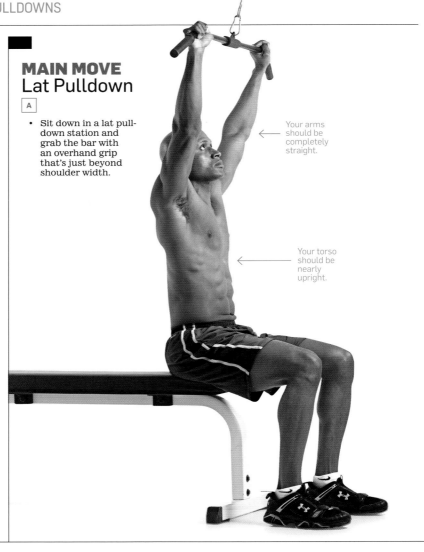

MAIN MOVE
Lat Pulldown

A

- Sit down in a lat pull-down station and grab the bar with an overhand grip that's just beyond shoulder width.

← Your arms should be completely straight.

← Your torso should be nearly upright.

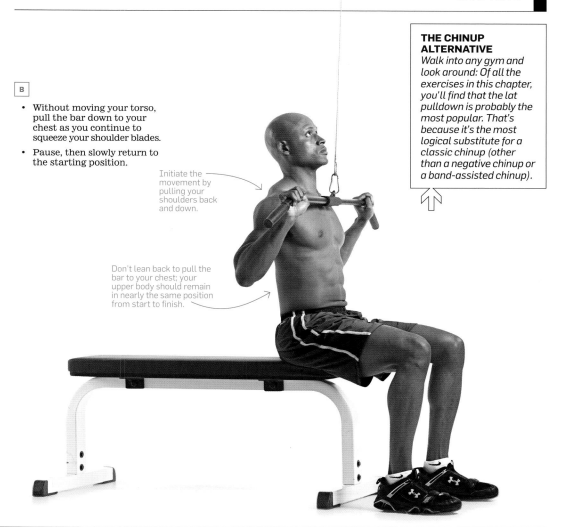

B

- Without moving your torso, pull the bar down to your chest as you continue to squeeze your shoulder blades.

- Pause, then slowly return to the starting position.

Initiate the movement by pulling your shoulders back and down.

Don't lean back to pull the bar to your chest; your upper body should remain in nearly the same position from start to finish.

THE CHINUP ALTERNATIVE
Walk into any gym and look around: Of all the exercises in this chapter, you'll find that the lat pulldown is probably the most popular. That's because it's the most logical substitute for a classic chinup (other than a negative chinup or a band-assisted chinup).

Lats | PULLDOWNS

VARIATION #1
Wide-Grip Lat Pulldown
• Use an overhand grip that's about 1½ times shoulder width.

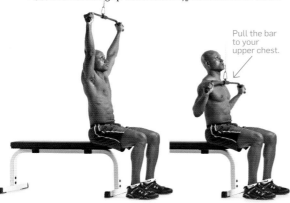

Pull the bar to your upper chest.

VARIATION #2
Underhand-Grip Lat Pulldown
• Use a shoulder-width, underhand grip.

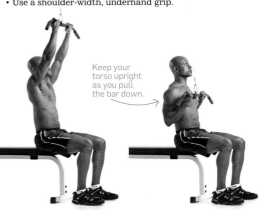

Keep your torso upright as you pull the bar down.

VARIATION #3
30-Degree Lat Pulldown

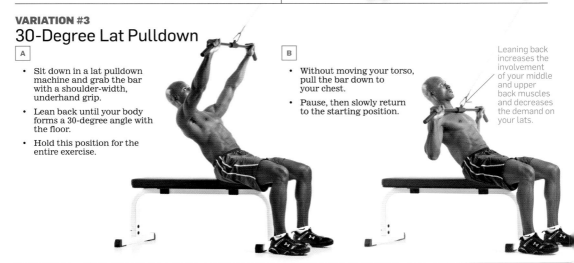

A

• Sit down in a lat pulldown machine and grab the bar with a shoulder-width, underhand grip.

• Lean back until your body forms a 30-degree angle with the floor.

• Hold this position for the entire exercise.

B

• Without moving your torso, pull the bar down to your chest.

• Pause, then slowly return to the starting position.

Leaning back increases the involvement of your middle and upper back muscles and decreases the demand on your lats.

THE BEST BACK EXERCISE YOU'VE NEVER DONE
Cable Face Pull with External Rotation

This unique movement simultaneously targets your upper back's scapular muscles and the rotator cuff muscles of your shoulders. Collectively, these muscles, which tend to be a weak spot in most guys, are the key to stable, healthy shoulders. As a result, the face pull with external rotation will help you avoid injuries and improve your upper-body strength. In fact, according to a survey of top *Men's Health* fitness advisors, this exercise is one of the best you can do.

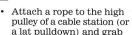
A

- Attach a rope to the high pulley of a cable station (or a lat pulldown) and grab an end with each hand.
- Back a few steps away from the weight stack until your arms are straight in front of you.

B

- Flare your elbows out, bend your arms, and pull the middle of the rope toward your eyes so your hands end up in line with your ears.
- Pause, then reverse back to the starting position.

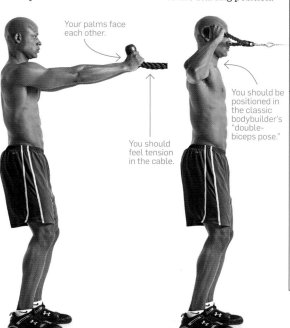

Your palms face each other.

You should feel tension in the cable.

You should be positioned in the classic bodybuilder's "double-biceps pose."

BONUS EXERCISE!

Lying Cable Face Pull with External Rotation

- If you can't maintain an upright posture while performing the cable face pull, try it while lying faceup on a flat bench.

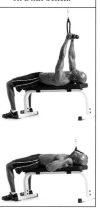

Shoulders

A great set of shoulders can work magic: They make your waist look slimmer, your arms look bigger, and your back look broader. And even better, they're among the easiest muscles for you to define, since the shoulder region is one of the last places your body deposits fat.

Plus, without strong shoulders, you're not likely to reach your full potential for size and strength in any of your other upper-body muscles. That's because your shoulders assist in most exercises for your chest, back, triceps, and biceps. So you might say they're your muscle-building MVP.

Bonus Benefits

An injury-proof upper body! Shoring up weaknesses in the muscles that surround your shoulder joints reduces your risk of a painful dislocation or rotator cuff tear.

Extra power! Whenever you throw or swing, your arms rotate from the shoulder joints. Strong shoulder muscles make it easier to move your arms with more power.

You'll stand taller! Weakness in the rotator cuff, the network of muscles on the back side of the shoulder joint, allows muscles on the front side of the joint to pull your shoulders forward, causing a slumped posture. But you can shift this balance of power by building a strong rotator cuff—so that you once again stand tall and proud.

Meet Your Muscles

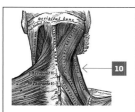

Levator Scapula
Most guys would consider the levator scapula [10] to be a neck muscle. And indeed, this ropelike muscle runs down the back of your neck and attaches to the inside edge of your shoulder blade. However, it works with your upper trapezius to help shrug your shoulder, which is why you can strengthen it with barbell and dumbbell shrugs.

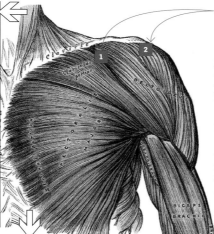

Deltoid
The roundish-looking muscle that caps the top of your upper arm is called your deltoid, and it's the shoulder muscle you're showing off when you wear a sleeveless shirt. It's made up of three distinct sections: your front deltoid [1], middle deltoid [2], and rear deltoid [3]. The best exercises for your front and middle delts are shoulder presses and shoulder raises. However, the top moves for working your rear deltoid are actually found in Chapter 2. That's because the same exercises that train the muscles of your middle and upper back are also the ones that work your rear delts.

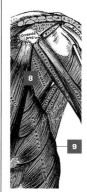

Serratus Anterior
Your serratus anterior [9] starts next to the outer edge of your pectorals, on the surface of your upper eight ribs. It wraps around your rib cage until it connects to the undersurface of your shoulder blade, along the inner edge. This muscle's job is to help stabilize and rotate your shoulder blade. You can make it stronger with the serratus shrug and the serratus chair shrug.

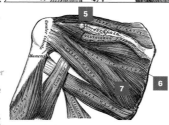

Rotator Cuff
Your rotator cuff muscles are a network of four muscles that attach your shoulder blade to your shoulder joint. They are the supraspinatus [5], the infraspinatus [6], the teres minor [7], and the subscapularis [8]. While these muscles are activated in just about every upper-body exercise—they contract to help stabilize your shoulder joint—they also need to be worked directly with shoulder rotation exercises.

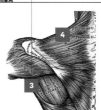

Upper Trapezius
Although the trapezius as a whole is categorized as a back muscle, the upper portions of your traps [4] are best developed with exercises such as the lateral raise and the shoulder shrug, both of which are featured in this chapter.

MUSCLE MISTAKE
Your Shoulders Hurt, but You Lift Anyway
Think of it this way: When your car gets a flat tire, you don't risk driving on it, since that could permanently damage the rims. It's the same way with your shoulders. But just avoiding the offending exercise isn't good enough. After all, a flat tire doesn't fix itself if you simply park the car in your garage. You need to take action. If you notice recurring shoulder pain, see an orthopedist or a physical therapist.

Shoulders |

In this chapter, you'll find 19 exercises that target the muscles of your shoulders. Throughout, you'll notice that certain exercises have been given the designation Main Move. Master this basic version of a movement, and you'll be able to do all of its variations with flawless form.

SHOULDER PRESSES

These exercises target your front deltoids, middle deltoids, and triceps. They also activate your upper traps, rotator cuff, and serratus anterior, which assist in the movement or act as stabilizers.

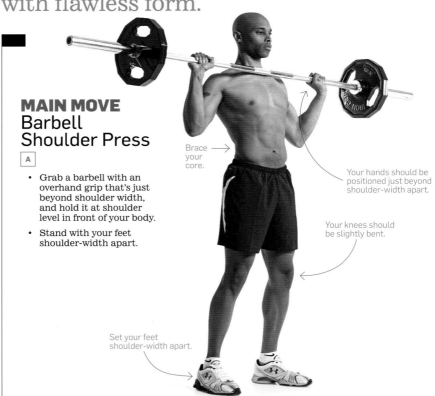

MAIN MOVE
Barbell Shoulder Press

A

- Grab a barbell with an overhand grip that's just beyond shoulder width, and hold it at shoulder level in front of your body.
- Stand with your feet shoulder-width apart.

Brace your core.

Your hands should be positioned just beyond shoulder-width apart.

Your knees should be slightly bent.

Set your feet shoulder-width apart.

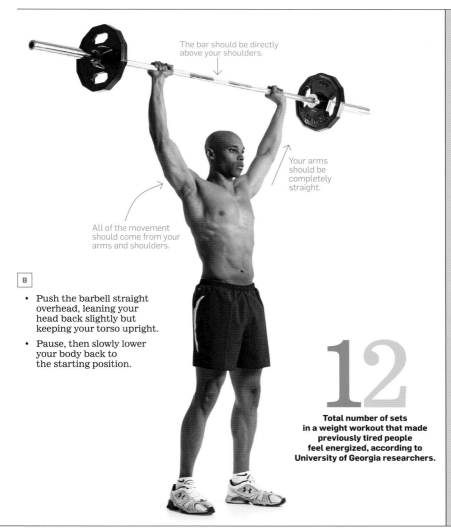

The bar should be directly above your shoulders.

Your arms should be completely straight.

All of the movement should come from your arms and shoulders.

B

- Push the barbell straight overhead, leaning your head back slightly but keeping your torso upright.

- Pause, then slowly lower your body back to the starting position.

12

Total number of sets in a weight workout that made previously tired people feel energized, according to University of Georgia researchers.

What about the Back Rest?

People often do the shoulder press seated, with their backs braced against a back rest. This provides a stable surface from which to lift, allowing the use of heavier weights. However, greater loads also mean increased stress on the shoulder joint in the "at-risk position"—the point at which your elbows are bent 90 degrees with your palms facing forward. This is the portion of the lift in which you're most likely to suffer a shoulder injury. Avoid that fate by skipping the back rest.

Shoulders | PRESSES

Barbell Push Press

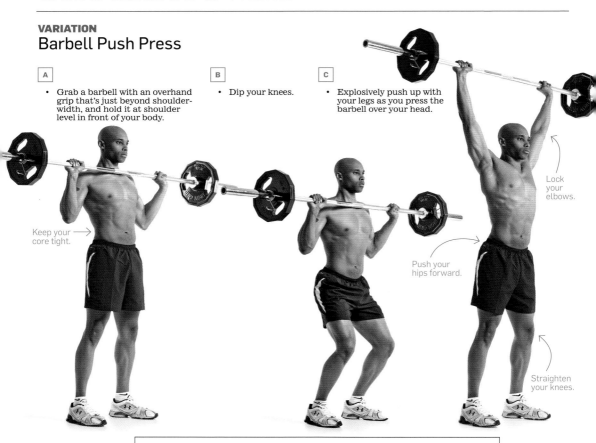

A

- Grab a barbell with an overhand grip that's just beyond shoulder-width, and hold it at shoulder level in front of your body.

B

- Dip your knees.

C

- Explosively push up with your legs as you press the barbell over your head.

Keep your core tight.

Push your hips forward.

Lock your elbows.

Straighten your knees.

MORE WEIGHT, LESS RISK

If you want to press heavier weights, try the push press. It doesn't carry the same injury risk as doing a shoulder press against a back rest (see "What about the Back Rest?" on the previous page). That's because your legs help you push through the at-risk position, reducing the strain on your shoulders.

MAIN MOVE
Dumbbell Shoulder Press

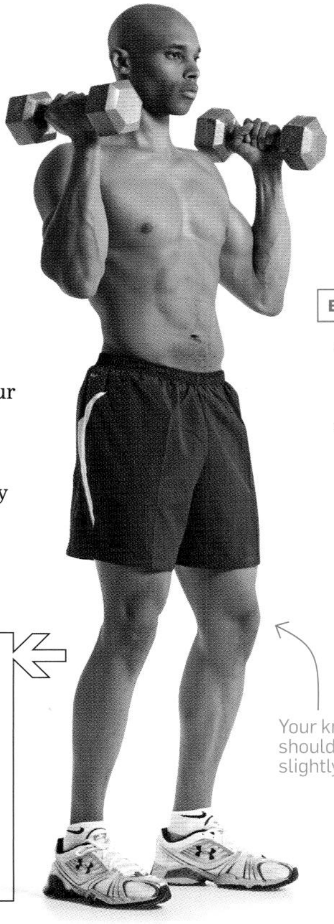

Push the dumbbells directly above your shoulders.

Lock your elbows.

Keep your core braced.

A

- Stand holding a pair of dumbbells just outside your shoulders, with your arms bent and palms facing each other.

- Set your feet shoulder-width apart, and slightly bend your knees.

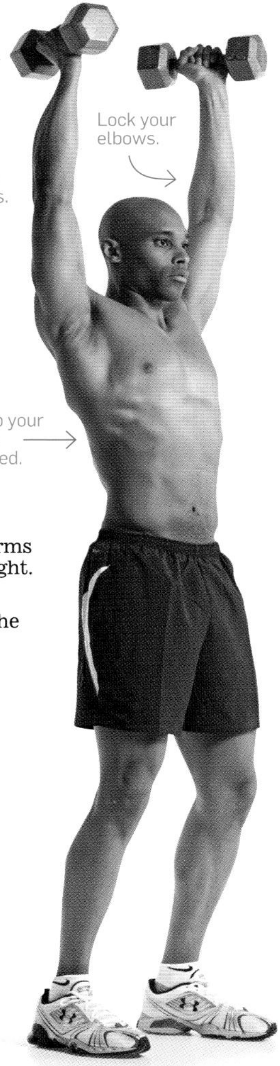

B

- Press the weights upward until your arms are completely straight.

- Slowly lower the dumbbells back to the starting position.

TRAINER'S TIP
Make sure to push the dumbbells in a straight line, rather than pushing them up and toward each other as many people do—a habit that increases the risk for shoulder injuries.

Your knees should be slightly bent.

Shoulders | PRESSES

VARIATION #1
Dumbbell Push Press

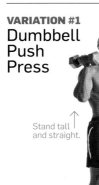

Stand tall and straight.

A

- Hold the dumbbells next to your shoulders with your elbows bent.

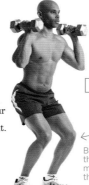

B

- Dip your knees.

Bend your knees so that you can generate more power to press the dumbbell.

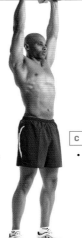

C

- Explosively push up with your legs as you press the dumbbells over your head.

VARIATION #2
Alternating Dumbbell Shoulder Press

A

- Hold the dumbbells next to your shoulders with your elbows bent.

Your palms should be facing each other.

Hold your core tight as you perform the exercise.

B

- Instead of pressing both dumbbells up at once, lift them one at a time, in an alternating fashion.

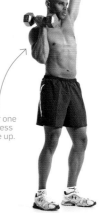

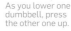

As you lower one dumbbell, press the other one up.

VARIATION #3
Seated Dumbbell Shoulder Press
• Sit at the end of a bench with your torso upright.

Your lower back should be naturally arched.

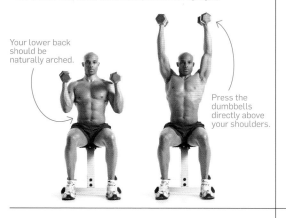

Press the dumbbells directly above your shoulders.

VARIATION #4
Swiss-Ball Dumbbell Shoulder Press
• Sit on a Swiss ball with your torso upright.

Your palms should be facing each other.

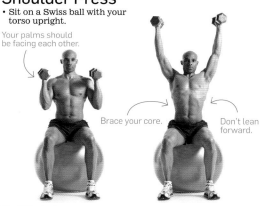

Brace your core.

Don't lean forward.

VARIATION #5
Alternating Swiss-Ball Dumbbell Shoulder Press
• Sit on a Swiss ball with your torso upright.

• Instead of pressing both dumbbells up at once, lift them one at a time, in an alternating fashion.

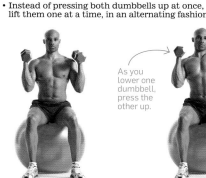
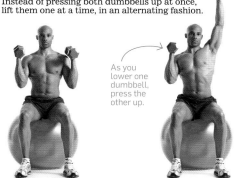

As you lower one dumbbell, press the other up.

VARIATION #6
Single-Arm Dumbbell Shoulder Press
• Perform a dumbbell shoulder press using only one dumbbell at a time.

• Complete the prescribed number of reps with your right arm, then immediately do the same number with your left arm.

Because using just one dumbbell causes uneven weight distribution across your body, this exercise increases the challenge to your core, making those muscles work harder to keep you balanced.

Let your free hand hang to your side or place it on your hip.

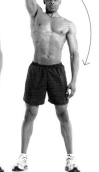

Shoulders | PRESSES

VARIATION #7
Dumbbell Alternating Shoulder Press and Twist

- Hold the dumbbells next to your shoulders with your elbows bent.

- Rotate your torso to the right as you press the dumbbell in your left hand at a slight angle above your shoulder.
- Reverse the movement back to the start, rotate to your left, and press the dumbbell in your right hand upward. Alternate back and forth.

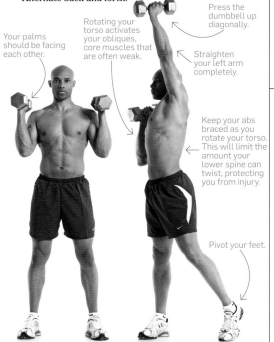

Your palms should be facing each other.

Rotating your torso activates your obliques, core muscles that are often weak.

Press the dumbbell up diagonally.

Straighten your left arm completely.

Keep your abs braced as you rotate your torso. This will limit the amount your lower spine can twist, protecting you from injury.

Pivot your feet.

Floor Inverted Shoulder Press

- Assume a pushup position, but move your feet forward and raise your hips so that your torso is nearly perpendicular to the floor.
- Your hands should be slightly wider than your shoulders, and your arms should be straight.
- Without changing your body posture, lower your body until your head nearly touches the floor.
- Pause, then return to the starting position by pushing your body back up until your arms are straight.

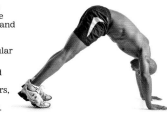

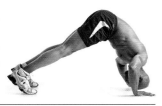

Inverted Shoulder Press

- Assume a pushup position, but place your feet on a bench and push your hips up so that your torso is nearly perpendicular to the floor.
- Without changing your body posture, lower your body until your head nearly touches the floor.

Your arms should be straight.

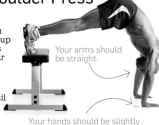

Your hands should be slightly wider than shoulder-width apart.

While the inverted shoulder press is technically a pushup, the tweak to your form shifts more of the workload to your shoulders and triceps, reducing the demand on your chest.

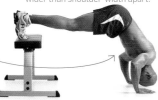

SHOULDER RAISES

These exercises target your front and middle deltoids. However, the different variations shift the section of the muscle that works the hardest. What's more, shoulder raises work your rear deltoids, upper traps, rotator cuff, and serratus anterior, since these muscles assist in raising the weight or act as stabilizers on nearly every version of this exercise.

MAIN MOVE
Front Raise

A

- Grab a pair of dumbbells and let them hang at arm's length next to your sides, with your palms facing each other.

B

- Raise your arms straight in front of you until they're parallel to the floor and perpendicular to your torso.
- Pause, then slowly lower the dumbbells back to the starting position.

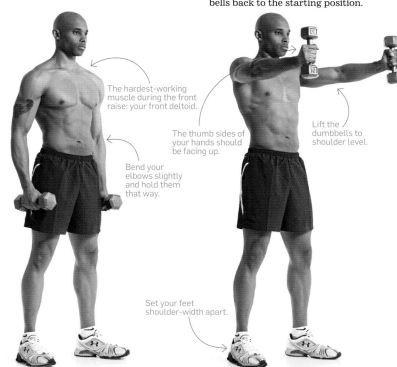

The hardest-working muscle during the front raise: your front deltoid.

The thumb sides of your hands should be facing up.

Lift the dumbbells to shoulder level.

Bend your elbows slightly and hold them that way.

Set your feet shoulder-width apart.

Shoulders | RAISES

MAIN MOVE
Lateral Raise

A

- Grab a pair of dumbbells and let them hang at arm's length next to your sides.
- Stand tall, with your feet shoulder-width apart.
- Turn your arms so that your palms are facing forward, and bend your elbows slightly.

B

- Without changing the bend in your elbows, raise your arms straight out to your sides until they're at shoulder level.
- Pause for 1 second at the top of the movement, then slowly lower the weights back to the starting position.

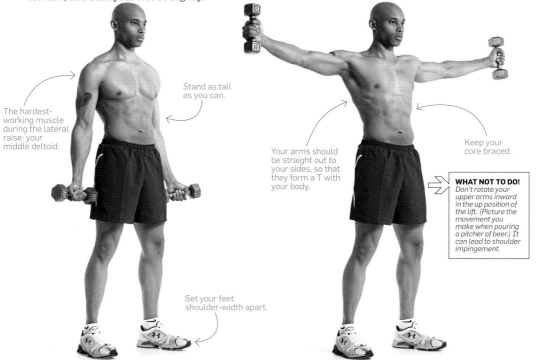

The hardest-working muscle during the lateral raise: your middle deltoid.

Stand as tall as you can.

Your arms should be straight out to your sides, so that they form a T with your body.

Keep your core braced.

WHAT NOT TO DO!
Don't rotate your upper arms inward in the up position of the lift. (Picture the movement you make when pouring a pitcher of beer.) It can lead to shoulder impingement.

Set your feet shoulder-width apart.

VARIATION #1
Alternating Lateral Raise with Static Hold

A

- Stand holding a pair of dumbbells straight out from your sides, as you would in the "up" position of a lateral raise.

B

- Lower and raise one arm, then lower and raise the other. That's one repetition.

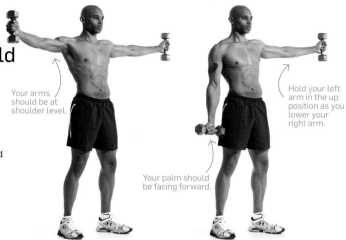

Your arms should be at shoulder level.

Hold your left arm in the up position as you lower your right arm.

Your palm should be facing forward.

VARIATION #2
Leaning Lateral Raise

A

- Hold a dumbbell in your left hand, at arm's length next to your side.
- Stand with your right leg next to a sturdy object such as a power rack.
- Place your left foot next to your right.
- Grab the power rack with your right hand and let your right arm straighten so that you're leaning to your left.

B

- Without changing the bend in your elbow, raise your left arm straight out to your side until it's at shoulder level.
- Lower and repeat.
- Complete the prescribed number of repetitions with your left arm, then immediately do the same number with your right arm.

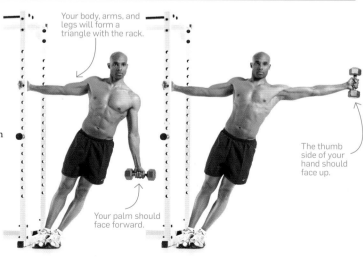

Your body, arms, and legs will form a triangle with the rack.

The thumb side of your hand should face up.

Your palm should face forward.

Shoulders | SHRUGS

MAIN MOVE
Dumbbell Shrug

- Grab a pair of dumbbells and let them hang at arm's length next to your sides, your palms facing each other.

- Shrug your shoulders as high as you can.
- Pause in the up position, then slowly lower the dumbbells back to the start.

To shrug, imagine that you're trying to touch your shoulders to your ears without moving any other parts of your body.

THE DUMBBELL ADVANTAGE?
Compared to the barbell shrug, the dumbbell shrug places less stress on your shoulder joints. That's because your shoulders don't have to rotate to hold the bar. This keeps them more stable as you perform the movement.

VARIATION
Overhead Dumbbell Shrug

- Hold a pair of dumbbells straight above your shoulders, with your arms completely straight and your palms facing out.

- Shrug your shoulders as high as you can.
- Pause, then reverse the movement back to the starting position.

Keep your arms straight.

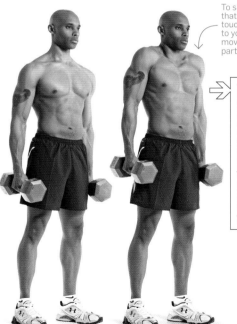

THE BEST SHOULDER EXERCISE YOU'VE NEVER DONE
Scaption and Shrug

This movement is the exercise that keeps on giving. That's because when you raise the dumbbells to perform scaption, you target your front deltoids, rotator cuff, and serratus anterior. Then comes the shrug. Like an overhead shrug, this version of the movement emphasizes your upper traps over your levator scapulae. This helps better balance the muscles that rotate your shoulder blades. The end result: Healthier shoulders and better posture.

A
- Stand holding a pair of dumbbells at arm's length next to your sides, your palms facing each other and your elbows slightly bent.

B
- Without changing the bend in your elbows, raise your arms at a 30-degree angle to your body (so that they form a Y) until they're at shoulder level.

C
- At the top of the movement, shrug your shoulders upward.

- Pause, then slowly lower the weight back to the starting position.

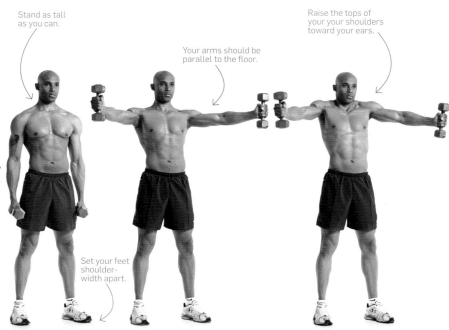

Stand as tall as you can.

Your arms should be parallel to the floor.

Raise the tops of your your shoulders toward your ears.

Set your feet shoulder-width apart.

Arms

Your arms are like built-in publicists for all the hard work you do in the gym. That's because they're the only major muscles you can expose almost anywhere, anytime. If your biceps and triceps are well-defined, people will assume the rest of you is chiseled as well.

The best part is that a sculpted set of arms isn't as hard to achieve as you might think. The reason: Just about every upper-body exercise—whether it's for your chest, back, or shoulders—also involves your arms. After all, these exercises require that you use your arms to help move the weights. So work hard on your other upper-body muscles, and your arms will benefit by default. Then you can simply use the specific biceps and triceps exercises in this chapter to give them a little extra love.

Bonus Benefits

Life is easier! Stronger biceps allow you to carry just about any object with less effort. So whether you're toting groceries or holding a baby, you'll notice the difference.

Damage control! Your triceps protect your elbow joints by acting as shock absorbers, lessening stress whenever your elbows are forced to flex suddenly, such as in breaking your fall in football or bracing yourself when mountain biking.

More muscle, everywhere! Your arms assist in exercises for all the muscles of your upper body. So if the smaller muscles of your arms give out too early, you'll be shortchanging the bigger muscles of your chest, back, and shoulders. Make sure your arms are strong, and you'll benefit all over.

Meet Your Muscles

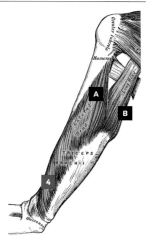

Biceps

The front of your upper arm owes its bulge to two muscle groups: your biceps brachii and your brachialis.

Your biceps brachii [1] originates at your shoulder and attaches to your forearm. Its duties are to bend your elbow and to rotate your forearm—a movement known as supination. Any type of arm curl works this muscle, as do chinups and rows.

Your brachialis [2] starts in the middle of your upper-arm bone and also attaches to your forearm. It assists your biceps brachii in bending your elbow.

The brachioradialis [3] originates on your upper-arm bone, near your elbow, and attaches close to your wrist. So it helps your biceps brachii bend your elbow and rotate your forearm, but it contributes little to the size of your biceps.

The biceps brachii is composed of two separate sections, or heads, that unite just before they attach to a forearm bone called the radius. The brachialis attaches to your ulna, the longer of the two forearm bones.

Triceps

The muscle on the back of your upper arm is called the triceps brachii [4]. When well-defined, it forms a horseshoe-like shape. Considering its name—triceps—it should be no surprise that the muscle is composed of three different sections, or heads. All three heads start on the back of either your upper arm or your shoulder blade, and then unite so that they attach together on your forearm. As a result, the primary job of your triceps is to straighten your arm. So this muscle is engaged in any exercise in which you straighten your arm against resistance: triceps extensions, triceps pressdowns and, of course, chest and shoulder presses.

The outer segment of your triceps is called the lateral head [A].

The middle segment of your triceps is called the medial head (not shown; hidden by the lateral head).

The inner segment of your triceps is called the long head [B].

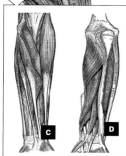

Forearms

Your wrist and finger flexors [C] are located on the inside of your forearm. They allow you to bend your wrist forward, and they can be trained with exercises such as wrist curls.

Your wrist extensors [D] are located on the outside, or "top," of your forearm. They allow you to bend your wrist backward, and they can be trained with exercises such as wrist extensions.

Biceps | ARM CURLS

In this chapter, you'll find 59 exercises that target the muscles of your arms. These exercises are divided between two major sections: Biceps and Triceps. Within each section, you'll notice that certain exercises have been given the designation Main Move. Master this basic version of a movement, and you'll be able to do all of its variations with flawless form.

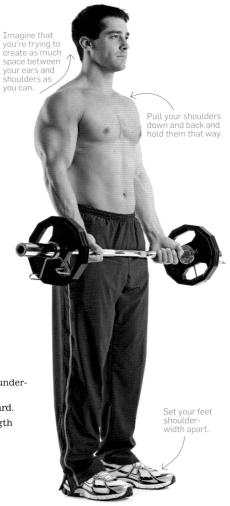

Imagine that you're trying to create as much space between your ears and shoulders as you can.

Pull your shoulders down and back and hold them that way.

Set your feet shoulder-width apart.

ARM CURLS
These exercises target your biceps brachii, brachialis, and brachioradialis. Your upper-back and rear-shoulder muscles also come into play, since they keep your shoulders stable as you curl a weight in front of your body.

MAIN MOVE
EZ-Bar Curl

A

- Grab an EZ-curl bar with an under-hand, shoulder-width grip.
- Your palms should angle inward.
- Let the bar hang at arm's length in front of your body.

2.5

Times more strength lifters gained when lowering a weight slowly and lifting it fast compared to performing each rep at a slow speed from start to finish, according to a George Washington University study.

Keep your chest up.

Stand as tall as you can for the entire exercise.

B

- Without moving your upper arms, bend your elbows and curl the bar as close to your shoulders as you can.

- Pause, then slowly lower the weight back to the starting position.

- Each time you return to the starting position, completely straighten your arms.

HOW DO YOU MEASURE UP?
Finding the circumferences of your arms is an excellent way to gauge the effectiveness of your arm workout. For the most accurate results, take all your measurements at the same time of day, such as before breakfast. (Your arms may be slightly larger after a workout or meal, when blood rushes to your muscles.) Extend your arm straight in front of you and wrap a measuring tape around the largest portion of your upper arm. Record the circumference, then measure your other arm.

Biceps | ARM CURLS

VARIATION #1
Close-Grip EZ-Bar Curl
- Hold the bar with a narrow underhand grip, your hands about 6 inches apart.

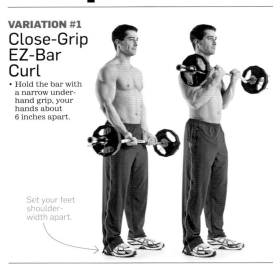

Set your feet shoulder-width apart.

VARIATION #2
Wide-Grip EZ-Bar Curl
- Hold the bar with an underhand grip that's about 1½ times shoulder width.

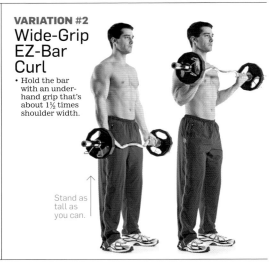

Stand as tall as you can.

VARIATION #3
Swiss-Ball Preacher Curl

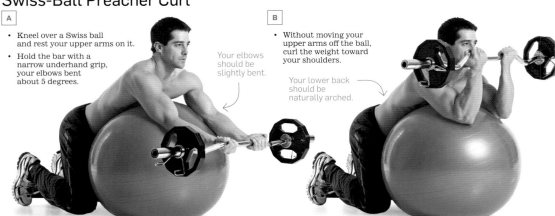

A
- Kneel over a Swiss ball and rest your upper arms on it.
- Hold the bar with a narrow underhand grip, your elbows bent about 5 degrees.

Your elbows should be slightly bent.

B
- Without moving your upper arms off the ball, curl the weight toward your shoulders.

Your lower back should be naturally arched.

VARIATION #4
EZ-Bar Preacher Curl

- Rest your upper arms on the sloping pad of a preacher bench and hold the bar in front of you, your elbows bent about 5 degrees.

- Without moving your upper arms, bend your elbows and curl the bar toward your shoulders.

Keep your upper arms on the pad.

Your hands should be about 6 inches apart.

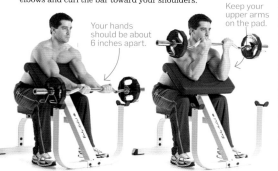

VARIATION #5
Reverse EZ-Bar Curl

- Hold the bar with an overhand, shoulder-width grip.

Your palms should be angled toward each other facing your thighs.

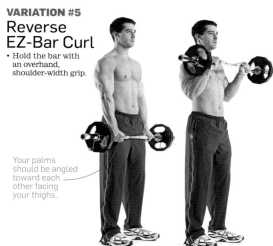

VARIATION #6
Telle Curl

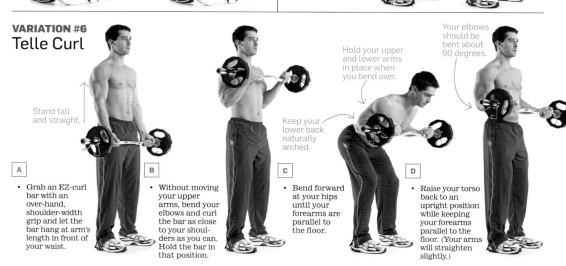

Stand tall and straight.

Hold your upper and lower arms in place when you bend over.

Keep your lower back naturally arched.

Your elbows should be bent about 90 degrees.

A
- Grab an EZ-curl bar with an over-hand, shoulder-width grip and let the bar hang at arm's length in front of your waist.

B
- Without moving your upper arms, bend your elbows and curl the bar as close to your shoulders as you can. Hold the bar in that position.

C
- Bend forward at your hips until your forearms are parallel to the floor.

D
- Raise your torso back to an upright position while keeping your forearms parallel to the floor. (Your arms will straighten slightly.)

Biceps | ARM CURLS

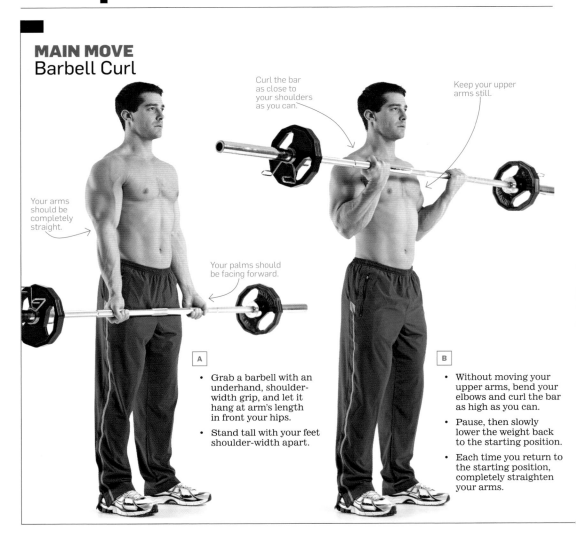

MAIN MOVE
Barbell Curl

Curl the bar as close to your shoulders as you can.

Keep your upper arms still.

Your arms should be completely straight.

Your palms should be facing forward.

A

- Grab a barbell with an underhand, shoulder-width grip, and let it hang at arm's length in front your hips.
- Stand tall with your feet shoulder-width apart.

B

- Without moving your upper arms, bend your elbows and curl the bar as high as you can.
- Pause, then slowly lower the weight back to the starting position.
- Each time you return to the starting position, completely straighten your arms.

VARIATION
Wide-Grip Barbell Curl

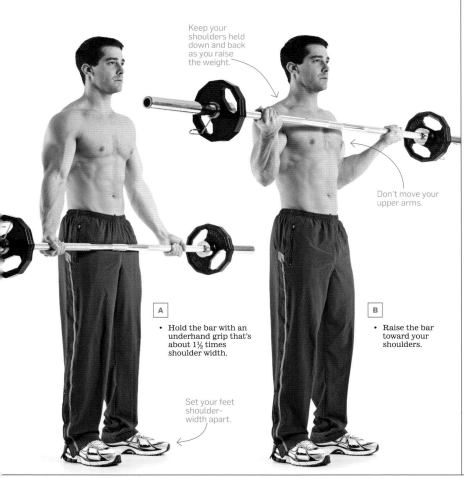

Keep your shoulders held down and back as you raise the weight.

Don't move your upper arms.

A
- Hold the bar with an underhand grip that's about 1½ times shoulder width.

Set your feet shoulder-width apart.

B
- Raise the bar toward your shoulders.

This is better known as "cheating." While this approach can allow you to lift heavier weights, it doesn't benefit your biceps. Colorado State University researchers found that leaning back and forth to complete a barbell curl simply transfers more of the workload to your shoulders. What's more, wildly swinging the weights up and down can damage the muscles, joints, and ligaments of your back. So stick to strict form.

Biceps | ARM CURLS

MAIN MOVE
Standing Dumbbell Curl

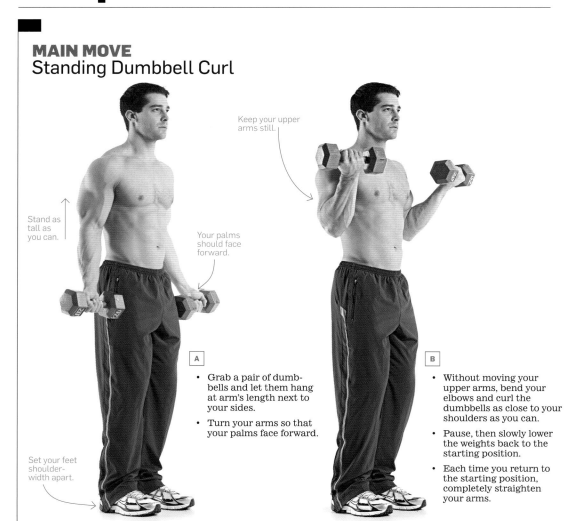

Keep your upper arms still.

Stand as tall as you can.

Your palms should face forward.

Set your feet shoulder-width apart.

A

- Grab a pair of dumbbells and let them hang at arm's length next to your sides.

- Turn your arms so that your palms face forward.

B

- Without moving your upper arms, bend your elbows and curl the dumbbells as close to your shoulders as you can.

- Pause, then slowly lower the weights back to the starting position.

- Each time you return to the starting position, completely straighten your arms.

VARIATION #1
Twisting Standing Dumbbell Curl

Besides using this method while standing, you also can use the twisting technique with any of the other body positions listed on the next page.

More Ways to Curl!

Instead of curling both dumbbells at once, lift them one at a time, in an alternating fashion. Simply raise and lower one dumbbell, then repeat with the other. You may be able to do more reps this way since one arm rests each time the other curls the dumbbell. So your biceps won't fatigue as fast. Another approach for variety: Simultaneously raise one dumbbell as you lower the other. You can use these techniques with any of the body positions and grips listed on the next page, as well as just about any other curl.

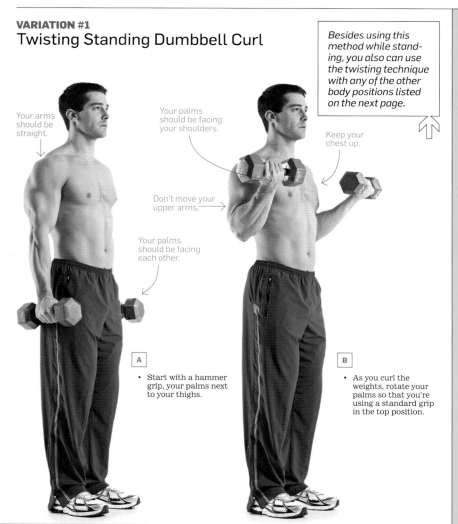

Your arms should be straight.

Your palms should be facing your shoulders.

Keep your chest up.

Don't move your upper arms.

Your palms should be facing each other.

A

- Start with a hammer grip, your palms next to your thighs.

B

- As you curl the weights, rotate your palms so that you're using a standard grip in the top position.

Biceps | ARM CURLS

VARIATIONS #2-25
Mix and match any of five grips with any of five body positions for 25 different variations of this exercise. Here, you'll see five examples of how the grips and body positions can be paired. But vary the combos frequently for best results.

BODY POSITION #1: INCLINE
Incline Offset-Thumb Dumbbell Curl

- Lie faceup on a bench that's set to a 45-degree incline.

- Lying on an incline causes your arms to hang behind your body, which emphasizes the long head of your biceps brachii to a greater degree.

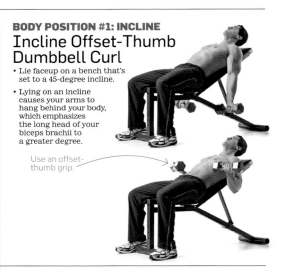

Use an offset-thumb grip.

BODY POSITION #2: DECLINE
Decline Hammer Curl

- Lie with your chest against a bench that's set to a 45-degree incline.

- This position causes your arms to hang in front of your body, placing more emphasis on your brachialis.

Don't move your upper arms.

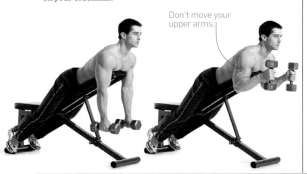

BODY POSITION #3: SEATED
Seated Reverse Dumbbell Curl

- Sit tall on a bench or Swiss ball.

- Performing the exercise in a seated position may make you less likely to rock your torso back and forth—or "cheat"—as you curl the weights.

Keep your chest up and your shoulders pulled down and back.

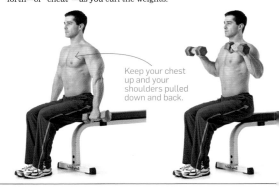

BODY POSITION #4: STANDING

Standing Dumbbell Curl

- Stand with your feet shoulder-width apart. (For complete instructions, see the standing dumbbell curl, also listed as the Main Move on page 76.)

- Anytime you're standing, you engage more core muscles than when you're sitting.

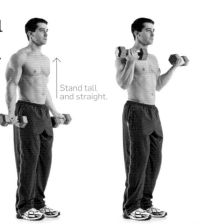

Stand tall and straight.

BODY POSITION #5: SPLIT STANCE

Split-Stance Offset-Pinky Dumbbell Curl

- Place one foot in front of you on a bench or step that's just higher than knee level.

- Putting one foot on a bench forces your hip and core muscles to work harder in order to keep your body stable.

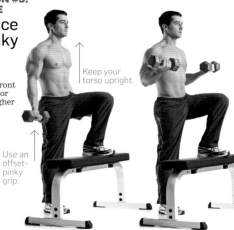

Keep your torso upright.

Use an offset-pinky grip.

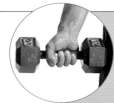

Standard Grip
Your palms face forward, and you grip the handle in the middle.
   This is the default dumbbell curl grip.

Offset-Pinky Grip
Your palms face forward, and each pinky finger touches the inside head of a dumbbell.
   This shifts the way the weight is distributed, providing more variety.

Offset-Thumb Grip
Your palms face forward, and each thumb touches the outside head of a dumbbell.
   This forces your biceps brachii to work harder to keep your forearm rotated outward as you curl the weight.

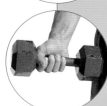

Hammer Grip
Your palms face each other.
   This causes your brachialis muscle to work harder for the entire movement.

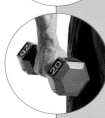

Reverse Grip
Your palms face behind you.
   This exercise targets your brachioradialis but decreases the activity of your biceps brachii. You'll really feel it in your forearms.

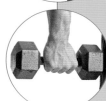

Biceps | ARM CURLS

VARIATION #26
Standing Zottman Curl

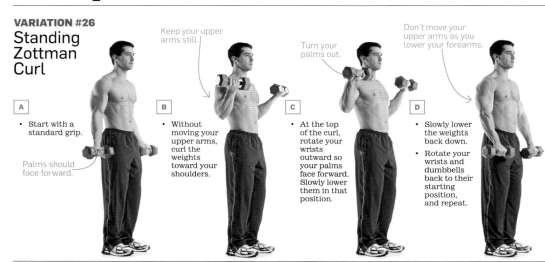

Keep your upper arms still.

Turn your palms out.

Don't move your upper arms as you lower your forearms.

A
- Start with a standard grip.

Palms should face forward.

B
- Without moving your upper arms, curl the weights toward your shoulders.

C
- At the top of the curl, rotate your wrists outward so your palms face forward. Slowly lower them in that position.

D
- Slowly lower the weights back down.
- Rotate your wrists and dumbbells back to their starting position, and repeat.

VARIATION #27
Static Curl

- Grab a dumbbell with your right hand and stand behind a raised incline bench.
- Place the back of your upper arm across the top of the bench.
- Lower the dumbbell until your arm is bent about 20 degrees.
- Hold that position for 40 seconds to build more muscle, or hold for 6 to 8 seconds for greater gains in strength. Then repeat with your left arm. That's one set.

PICK THE RIGHT WEIGHT *Choose the heaviest dumbbell that allows you to hold for the length of time that matches your goal. So if you're building strength, you'll use a heavier weight than if you're focusing on faster muscle growth.*

The mid-part of your upper arm should be the only part touching the bench.

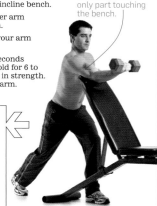

VARIATION #28
Dumbbell Curl with Static Hold

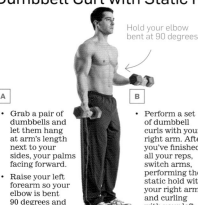

Hold your elbow bent at 90 degrees.

A
- Grab a pair of dumbbells and let them hang at arm's length next to your sides, your palms facing forward.
- Raise your left forearm so your elbow is bent 90 degrees and hold it there.

B
- Perform a set of dumbbell curls with your right arm. After you've finished all your reps, switch arms, performing the static hold with your right arm and curling with your left.

80

VARIATION #29
Hammer Curl to Press

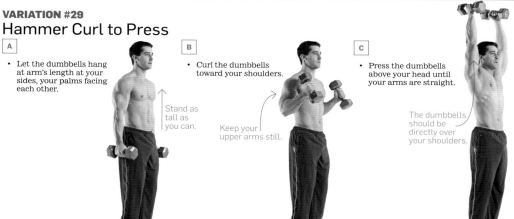

A
- Let the dumbbells hang at arm's length at your sides, your palms facing each other.

Stand as tall as you can.

B
- Curl the dumbbells toward your shoulders.

Keep your upper arms still.

C
- Press the dumbbells above your head until your arms are straight.

The dumbbells should be directly over your shoulders.

VARIATION #30
Split-Stance Hammer Curl to Press

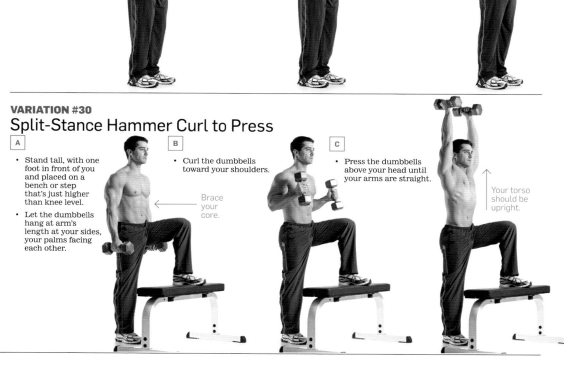

A
- Stand tall, with one foot in front of you and placed on a bench or step that's just higher than knee level.
- Let the dumbbells hang at arm's length at your sides, your palms facing each other.

Brace your core.

B
- Curl the dumbbells toward your shoulders.

C
- Press the dumbbells above your head until your arms are straight.

Your torso should be upright.

Triceps | ARM EXTENSIONS

MAIN MOVE
Dumbbell Lying Triceps Extension

A

- Grab a pair of dumbbells and lie faceup on a flat bench.
- Hold the dumbbells over your head with straight arms, your palms facing each other.

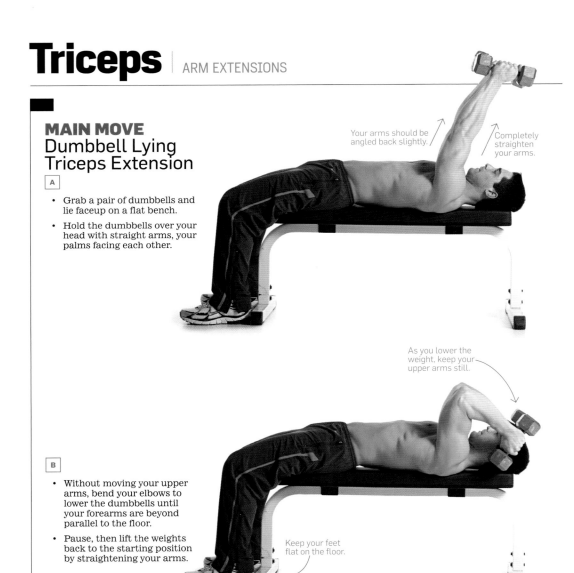

Your arms should be angled back slightly.

Completely straighten your arms.

As you lower the weight, keep your upper arms still.

B

- Without moving your upper arms, bend your elbows to lower the dumbbells until your forearms are beyond parallel to the floor.
- Pause, then lift the weights back to the starting position by straightening your arms.

Keep your feet flat on the floor.

VARIATION #1
Alternating Dumbbell Lying Triceps Extension

Your arms should be angled back slightly.

- Grab a pair of dumbbells and lie on your back on a flat bench, with your palms facing each other and your arms straight.

- Instead of lowering both dumbbells at once, lower them one at a time, in an alternating fashion.

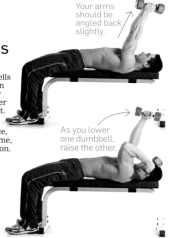

As you lower one dumbbell, raise the other.

VARIATION #2
Swiss-Ball Dumbbell Lying Triceps Extension

- Instead of lying on a flat bench, perform the movement with your middle and upper back placed firmly on a Swiss ball, and raise your hips so they're in line with your torso.

- Without moving your upper arms, bend your elbows to lower the dumbbells until your forearms are beyond parallel to the floor.

Your body should form a straight line from your shoulders to your knees.

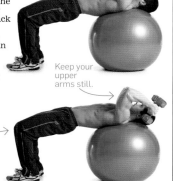

Keep your upper arms still.

VARIATION #3
Lying Dumbbell Pullover to Extension

A

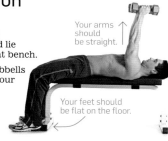

- Grab a pair of dumbbells and lie faceup on a flat bench.

- Hold the dumbbells directly over your shoulders.

- Your palms should be facing each other.

Your arms should be straight.

Your feet should be flat on the floor.

B

- Without moving your upper arms, bend your elbows to lower the dumb-bells until your forearms are parallel to the floor.

Your elbows should be bent 90 degrees.

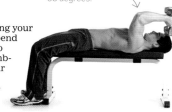

C

- Without changing the bend in your elbows, lower the dumbbells back beyond your head as far as you comfortably can.

- Pause, then reverse through each phase of the movement, back to the starting position.

Your elbows should stay bent 90 degrees as you lower your upper arms.

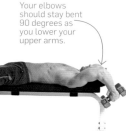

Triceps | ARM EXTENSIONS

MAIN MOVE
Dumbbell Overhead Triceps Extension

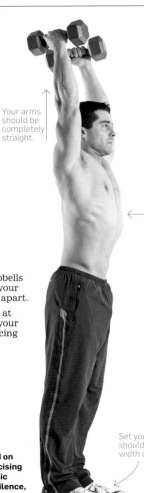

Your arms should be completely straight.

← Brace your core.

A

- Grab a pair of dumbbells and stand tall with your feet shoulder-width apart.

- Hold the dumbbells at arm's length above your head, your palms facing each other.

2

Times better people did on cognitive tests after exercising while listening to music compared to sweating in silence, according to an Ohio State University study.

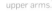
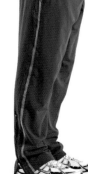

Your forearms should be at least parallel to the floor.

Don't move your upper arms.

B

- Without moving your upper arms, lower the dumbbells behind your head.

- Pause, then straighten your arms to return the dumbbells to the starting position.

Set your feet shoulder-width apart.

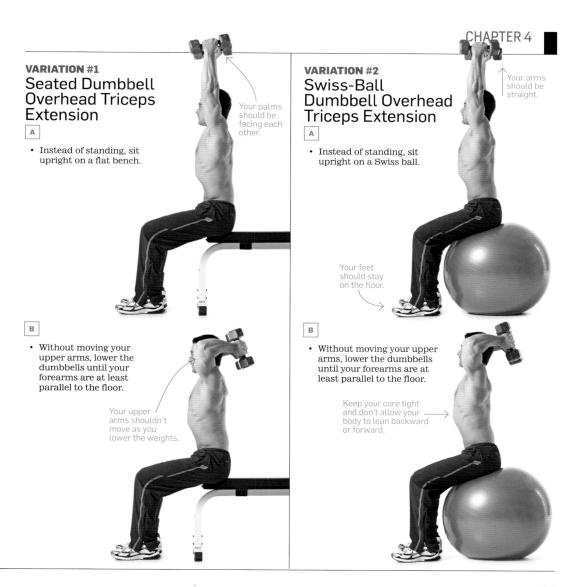

VARIATION #1
Seated Dumbbell Overhead Triceps Extension

A

- Instead of standing, sit upright on a flat bench.

Your palms should be facing each other.

B

- Without moving your upper arms, lower the dumbbells until your forearms are at least parallel to the floor.

Your upper arms shouldn't move as you lower the weights.

VARIATION #2
Swiss-Ball Dumbbell Overhead Triceps Extension

A

- Instead of standing, sit upright on a Swiss ball.

Your arms should be straight.

Your feet should stay on the floor.

B

- Without moving your upper arms, lower the dumbbells until your forearms are at least parallel to the floor.

Keep your core tight and don't allow your body to lean backward or forward.

Triceps | ARM EXTENSIONS

MAIN MOVE
Triceps Pressdown

TRAINER'S TIP
*If you use too much
weight in the triceps
pressdown, you'll
involve your back and
shoulder muscles,
defeating the pur-
pose. One strategy to
avoid that mistake:
Imagine you're
wearing tight
suspenders that hold
your shoulders down
as you do the exer-
cise. Can't keep them
down? You need to
use a lighter weight.*

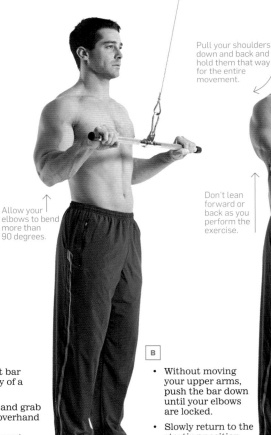

Pull your shoulders
down and back and
hold them that way
for the entire
movement.

Allow your
elbows to bend
more than
90 degrees.

Don't lean
forward or
back as you
perform the
exercise.

A

- Attach a straight bar
  to the high pulley of a
  cable station.
- Bend your arms and grab
  the bar with an overhand
  grip, your hands
  shoulder-width apart.
- Tuck your upper arms
  next to your sides.

B

- Without moving
  your upper arms,
  push the bar down
  until your elbows
  are locked.
- Slowly return to the
  starting position.

86

VARIATION #1
Underhand-Grip Triceps Pressdown
- Hold the bar with an underhand grip.

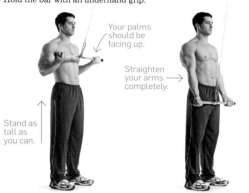

Your palms should be facing up.

Straighten your arms completely. →

Stand as tall as you can.

VARIATION #2
Rope Triceps Pressdown
- Hold an end of the rope with each hand.

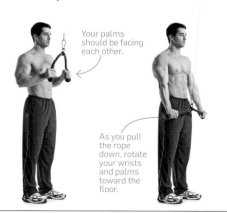

Your palms should be facing each other.

As you pull the rope down, rotate your wrists and palms toward the floor.

VARIATION #3
Single-Arm Rope Triceps Pressdown

A

- Hold an end of the rope with your right hand, your palm facing in.

B

- Complete the prescribed number of reps with your right arm, then immediately do the same number with your left arm.

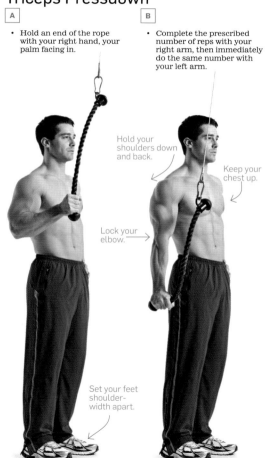

Hold your shoulders down and back.

Keep your chest up.

Lock your elbow. →

Set your feet shoulder-width apart.

Arms

THE BEST ARM EXERCISES YOU'VE NEVER DONE
Triple-Stop EZ-Bar Curl

What makes these moves so special? They require you to stop for 10 seconds at three different positions as you perform the movement. Pausing at each point increases strength at that joint angle and 10 degrees in either direction. So this helps eliminate any weak points you might have. It also keeps your muscles under tension for more than 30 seconds each set, a key for building muscle. You can apply the technique to nearly any variation of the arm curl or arm extension.

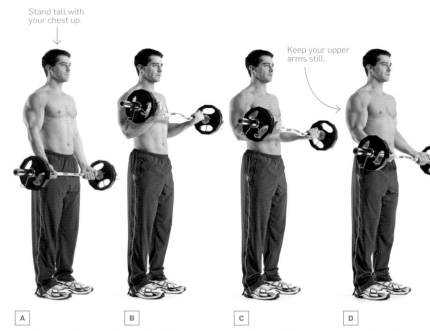

Stand tall with your chest up.

Keep your upper arms still.

A

• Do an EZ-bar curl, but as you lower the bar, pause for 10 seconds each at the three positions shown. One complete repetition is one set.

B

• First stop: You've lowered the bar about 2 inches.

C

• Second stop: Your elbows are bent 90 degrees.

D

• Third stop: A couple of inches before your arms are straight.

Triple-Stop Lying Dumbbell Triceps Extension

- Do a lying dumbbell triceps extension, but pause for 10 seconds each at the three positions shown. One complete repetition is one set.

- First stop: You've lowered the weights about 4 inches.

- Second stop: Your elbows are bent about 90 degrees.

- Lower the weights to the bottom position of the exercise.

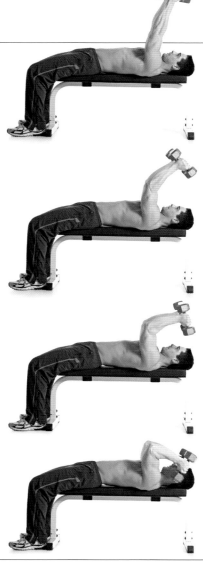

Quads
& Calves

I t can be tempting to skip exercises that work your quadriceps. No doubt this is because the movements that best train these muscles—squats and lunges—require a lot of effort. But, of course, that's exactly what makes them so worthwhile. Take the squat, for example. It burns more calories per rep than almost any other exercise. And along with targeting your quadriceps, it hits all the other muscles in your lower body, too, including your hamstrings, glutes, and calves.

So sure, squats and lunges are hard, but embracing the quadriceps exercises in this chapter will reward you with strong, muscular legs and a leaner midsection. And for those who want to give their lower legs extra attention, this section also includes moves that focus *directly* on your calves.

Bonus Benefits

Great abs! Besides helping you burn belly flab, squats work the muscles of your core harder than many ab exercises do.

Stronger back! In a study of lifters who did both upper- and lower-body exercises, Norwegian scientists found that those who emphasized lower-body movements such as the squat and lunge gained the most upper-body strength.

Better balance! Conditioning your quads also strengthens the ligaments and tendons within your legs—helping make your knees more stable and less susceptible to injury.

Meet Your Muscles

Quadriceps

The main muscles on the front of your thigh are your quadriceps [1]. This muscle group has four distinct sections: the rectus femoris [A], vastus lateralis [B], vastus medialis [C], and vastus intermedius [not shown; hidden beneath the rectus femoris]. All of these segments come together at the quadriceps tendon [D] and attach just below your knee joint. As a whole, their main function is to straighten your knee. That's why squats and lunges are the best exercises for working your quadriceps: They require that you straighten your legs against a resistance, even if it's just your body weight.

Gastrocnemius

Your calf consists of two separate muscles, both located on the back of your lower leg. The muscle closest to the surface of the skin is called the gastrocnemius [3]. It's composed of two sections—one on the inside of your leg, the other on the outside. These sections start just above your knee and come together at your Achilles tendon [4], which attaches to the back of your heel.

Hip Adductors

Your hip adductors [2] are the muscles on the inside of your thigh, or what's typically referred to as your groin. When your leg is straight out to the side, your hip adductors allow you to pull it back toward your body, a movement known as "hip adduction." (Creative name, huh?) These muscles are heavily involved in squats and lunges.

Soleus

Your other calf muscle, the soleus [5], lies underneath your gastrocnemius. It starts just below your knee and joins up with the gastrocnemius at your Achilles tendon. The primary duty of both calf muscles is to extend your ankle. Think of this as the action of raising your heel when your foot is flat on the floor. So besides calf raises, any exercise that features some level of ankle extension—such as the squats or jumping movements—also work your calf muscles.

Quads & Calves |

In this chapter, you'll find 59 exercises that target the muscles of your front thighs and lower legs. Throughout, you'll notice that certain exercises have been given the designation Main Move. Master this basic version of a movement, and you'll be able to do all of its variations with flawless form.

SQUATS

These exercises target your quadriceps. They also activate your core and just about every other muscle of your lower body, including your glutes, hamstrings, and calves. This makes the squat one of the best all-around exercises you can do.

MAIN MOVE
Body-Weight Squat

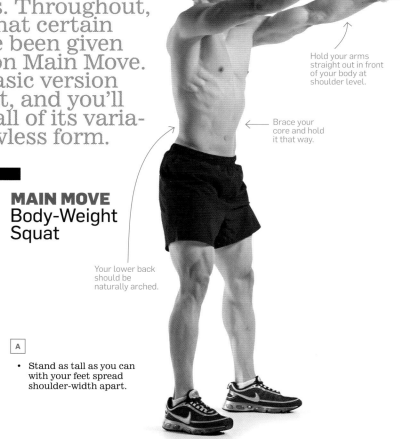

Hold your arms straight out in front of your body at shoulder level.

Brace your core and hold it that way.

Your lower back should be naturally arched.

A

- Stand as tall as you can with your feet spread shoulder-width apart.

1,250

Most weight, in pounds, ever squatted in competition.

SET YOUR STANCE
Jump as high as you can three times in a row. Then look down at your foot placement. This is roughly where you want to place your feet when you squat.

⇑

Your arms should stay in the same position from start to finish.

Your torso should stay as upright as possible.

Don't let your lower back round.

Keep your core tight.

The tops of your thighs should be parallel to the floor or lower.

Keep your weight on your heels, not on your toes, for the entire movement. One gauge: If your weight is distributed correctly, you should be able to wiggle your toes at any moment during the lift.

B

- Lower your body as far as you can by pushing your hips back and bending your knees.

- Pause, then slowly push yourself back to the starting position.

The Secret to a Perfect Squat

Hone your squat technique with this muscle-memory trick from Mel Siff, PhD, author of *Supertraining* and one of the all-time great minds in the field of exercise science. It's an easy way to help your body and brain learn the proper movement of the lift.

What to do: Prior to your first set of squats, sit tall on a bench with your back upright and naturally arched, your shoulders pulled back, and your lower legs perpendicular to the floor and at least shoulder-width apart. Hold your arms straight out in front of your body at shoulder level so that they're parallel to the floor. Bend forward at your hips—without changing the arch in your back—and move your feet back toward you just enough that you're able to stand up slowly, without having to rock backward or forward or change your body posture. Pay attention: That's the position you should be in when you squat. Once standing, reverse the movement and slowly lower your body to the seated position. Repeat several times.

Quads & Calves | SQUATS

VARIATION #1
Prisoner Squat

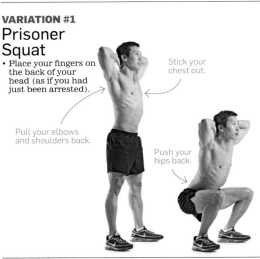

- Place your fingers on the back of your head (as if you had just been arrested).

Pull your elbows and shoulders back.

Stick your chest out.

Push your hips back.

VARIATION #2
Body-Weight Squat with Knee Press-Out

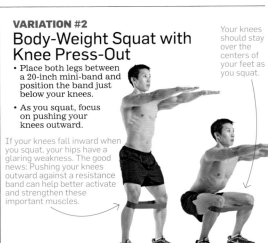

- Place both legs between a 20-inch mini-band and position the band just below your knees.

- As you squat, focus on pushing your knees outward.

If your knees fall inward when you squat, your hips have a glaring weakness. The good news: Pushing your knees outward against a resistance band can help better activate and strengthen these important muscles.

Your knees should stay over the centers of your feet as you squat.

VARIATION #3
Body-Weight Wall Squat

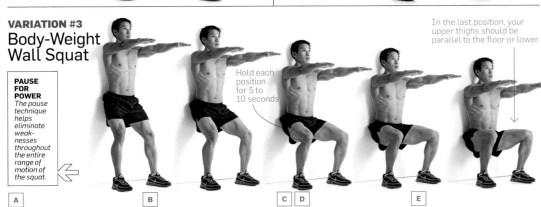

PAUSE FOR POWER
The pause technique helps eliminate weaknesses throughout the entire range of motion of the squat.

Hold each position for 5 to 10 seconds

In the last position, your upper thighs should be parallel to the floor or lower.

A

B

C D

E

- Lean back against a wall, with your feet about 2 feet away from it and shoulder-width apart.

- Keeping your back against the wall, bend your knees slightly so that your body descends a few inches. Hold for 5 to 10 seconds.

- Continue to lower yourself a few inches at a time, four more times.

- Once you've paused at all five positions, stand up and rest. That's one set.

VARIATION #4
Swiss-Ball Body-Weight Wall Squat

A

- Hold a Swiss ball behind you and stand so that the ball is pinned between your back and the wall.

- Place your feet about 2 feet in front of your body.

B

- Keeping your back in contact with the ball, lower your body until your upper thighs are at least parallel to the floor.

THE BEGINNER'S SQUAT
If you have trouble doing a standard body-weight squat, try the Swiss-ball version. It requires less core strength, which makes the exercise easier while helping you learn perfect form.

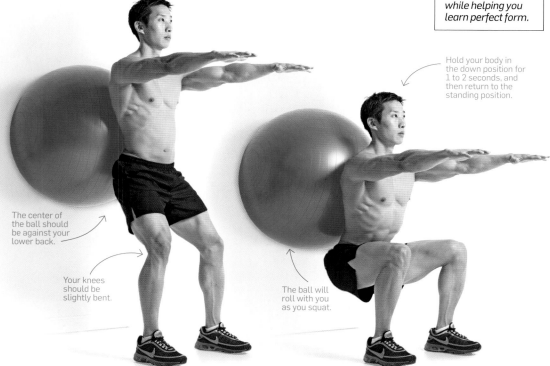

The center of the ball should be against your lower back.

Your knees should be slightly bent.

Hold your body in the down position for 1 to 2 seconds, and then return to the standing position.

The ball will roll with you as you squat.

Quads & Calves | SQUATS

VARIATION #5
Body-Weight Jump Squat

A

- Place your fingers on the back of your head and pull your elbows back so that they're in line with your body.

> **SQUAT FOR FAT LOSS**
> *While the jump squat variation shown here is great for athletic performance, use a deeper squat when doing the exercise for fat loss. In fact, lower your body until your upper thighs are parallel to the floor (as shown in the iso-explosive body-weight jump squat below).*

B

- Dip your knees in preparation to leap.

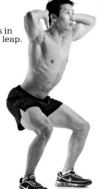

C

- Explosively jump as high as you can.
- When you land, immediately squat down and jump again.

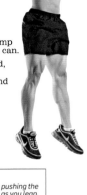

> **JUMP HIGHER**
> *Imagine that you're pushing the floor away from you as you leap.*

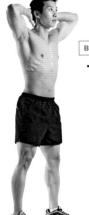

VARIATION #6
Iso-Explosive Body-Weight Jump Squat

- Place your fingers on the back of your head and pull your elbows back so that they're in line with your body.
- Push your hips back, bend your knees, and lower until your upper thighs are parallel to the floor.
- Pause for 5 seconds in the down position.
- After your pause, jump as high as you can.
- Land and reset.

> **WORK YOUR LEGS ANYWHERE**
> *The 5-second pause during this exercise eliminates all the elasticity in your muscles, which allows you to activate a maximum number of muscle fibers as you push yourself off the floor. This makes it a great exercise to use when you don't have access to weights.*

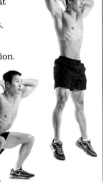

VARIATION #7
Braced Squat

- Hold a weight plate in front of your chest with both hands, your arms completely straight.

The braced squat overloads your core, helping to improve stability, strength, and performance. It's categorized as a body-weight exercise because the amount of weight you can use is limited due to shoulder fatigue from holding the plate in front of your body.

> **BUILD YOUR BICEPS, TOO!**
> *As you perform the braced squat, you can work your arms by doing a curl at the top of each repetition. With your arms outstretched, simply curl the plate toward your shoulders without moving your upper arms. Straighten your arms as you lower your body.*

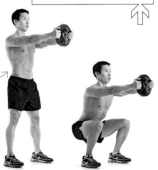

High Box Jump

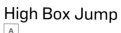

- Stand in front of a sturdy, secure box that's high enough so that you have to jump with great effort in order to land on top of it.

- Your feet should be shoulder-width apart.

- Dip your knees.

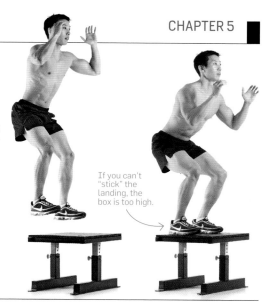

B **C**

- Jump up onto the box with a soft landing.

- Step down and reset your feet.

If you can't "stick" the landing, the box is too high.

Depth Jump

A

- Stand at the edge of a 12-inch box.

ADD INCHES TO YOUR VERTICAL
The depth jump is one of the best drills for improving your vertical leap. Try it twice a week, doing four or five sets of three repetitions at the beginning of your workout. Rest for 60 to 90 seconds between sets.

B

- Simply step off the box so that you land on both feet simultaneously (balls of feet first, followed by heels).

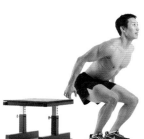

C

- When you make contact with the floor, jump as high as you can. That's one repetition.

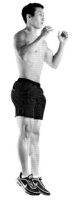

Quads & Calves | SQUATS

MAIN MOVE
Single-Leg Squat

A

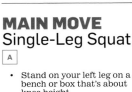

- Stand on your left leg on a bench or box that's about knee height.
- Hold your arms straight out in front of you.

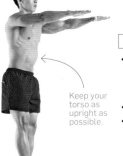

Keep your torso as upright as possible.

Flex your right ankle so that your toes are higher than your heel.

B

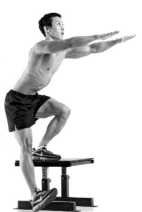

- Balancing on your left foot, bend your left knee and slowly lower your body until your right heel lightly touches the floor.
- Pause, then push yourself up.
- Complete the prescribed number of reps with your left leg, then immediately do the same number with your right.
- If this exercise is too hard, try the partial single-leg squat or the single-leg bench getup.

VARIATION #1
Single-Leg Bench Getup

A

- Sit tall on a bench with your back upright and naturally arched.
- Hold your arms straight out in front of your body at shoulder level, parallel to the floor.
- Raise your left foot off the floor.

Your lower back should be naturally arched.

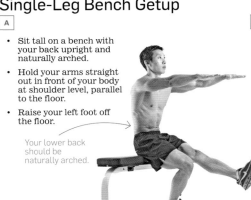

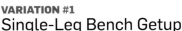

B

- Without leaning foward, press your body to a standing position. (If you can't do this, try sliding your foot slightly back toward your body in the starting position.)
- Sit back down.

Push your hips forward.

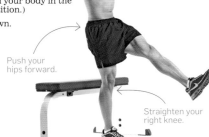

Straighten your right knee.

VARIATION #2
Partial Single-Leg Squat

A

- Stand on your left leg on a bench or box that's about knee height.
- Hold your arms straight out in front of you.

Flex your right ankle so that your toes are higher than your heel.

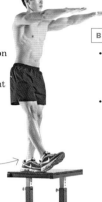

B

- Lower your body to just above your breaking point (see "Find Your Breaking Point" at right).
- Pause for 2 seconds before you push yourself back to a standing position.

To return to the start, press your left heel into the step and forcefully drive your body upward.

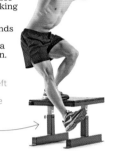

VARIATION #3
Pistol Squat

A

- Stand holding your arms straight out in front of your body at shoulder level, parallel to the floor.
- Raise your right leg off the floor, and hold it there.

Brace your core.

Your right leg should be straight.

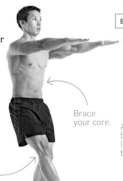

B

- Push your hips back and lower your body as far as you can.
- Pause, then push your body back to the starting position.

Keep your torso as upright as possible.

As you lower your body, raise your right leg so that it doesn't touch the floor.

Find Your Breaking Point

If you can't do at least three reps of the single-leg squat, try the partial single-leg squat. You'll first need to identify your breaking point. Your breaking point is the position you're in when you can no longer control the speed at which you lower your body. This could be after you've lowered yourself just an inch, or it could be after several inches. Determine its location, then follow the directions for the partial single-leg squat. As your strength improves, your breaking point will move lower. So retest it regularly.

Quads & Calves | SQUATS

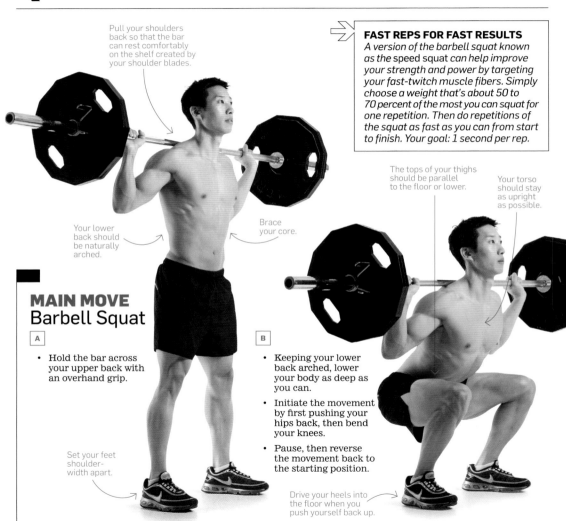

Pull your shoulders back so that the bar can rest comfortably on the shelf created by your shoulder blades.

Your lower back should be naturally arched.

Brace your core.

The tops of your thighs should be parallel to the floor or lower.

Your torso should stay as upright as possible.

FAST REPS FOR FAST RESULTS
A version of the barbell squat known as the speed squat can help improve your strength and power by targeting your fast-twitch muscle fibers. Simply choose a weight that's about 50 to 70 percent of the most you can squat for one repetition. Then do repetitions of the squat as fast as you can from start to finish. Your goal: 1 second per rep.

MAIN MOVE
Barbell Squat

A

- Hold the bar across your upper back with an overhand grip.

Set your feet shoulder-width apart.

B

- Keeping your lower back arched, lower your body as deep as you can.

- Initiate the movement by first pushing your hips back, then bend your knees.

- Pause, then reverse the movement back to the starting position.

Drive your heels into the floor when you push yourself back up.

VARIATION #1
Wide-Stance Barbell Squat

A

- Perform a squat with your feet set at twice shoulder width.

If your heels rise off the floor when you do a standard barbell squat, your hips are tight. But the wide-stance version of the exercise can help. Simply lower your body into the deepest position of the wide-stance squat that you can without allowing your heels to rise. Hold for 2 seconds. Try to lower your body a little farther with each workout. As your flexibility improves, narrow your stance and decrease the angle at which your toes point out.

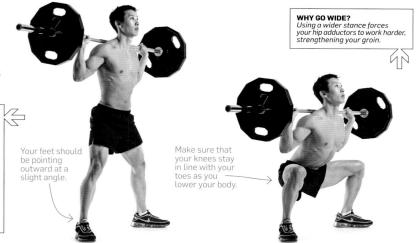

Your feet should be pointing outward at a slight angle.

Make sure that your knees stay in line with your toes as you lower your body.

WHY GO WIDE?
Using a wider stance forces your hip adductors to work harder, strengthening your groin.

VARIATION #2
Barbell Front Squat

A

- Hold the bar with an overhand grip that's just beyond shoulder width.
- Raise your upper arms until they're parallel to the floor.
- Allow the bar to roll back so that it's resting on the fronts of your shoulders.

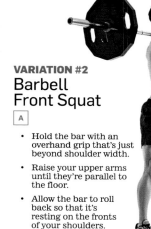

B

- Slowly lower your body until the tops of your thighs are at least parallel to the floor.
- Pause, then push your body back to the starting position.

Set your feet shoulder-width apart.

Keep your upper arms parallel to the floor for the entire movement. This prevents the bar from rolling forward and also helps you maintain a more upright posture.

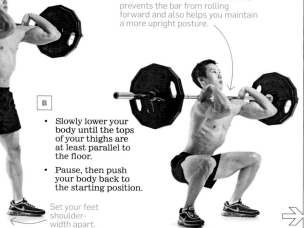

STRAPS
If your wrists aren't flexible enough to perform the traditional version of the barbell front squat, use this trick: Loop a pair of wrist straps around the bar—spaced shoulder-width apart—and cinch them tight. Then grasp the straps instead of bending your wrists back and resting the bar on your fingers.

Quads & Calves | SQUATS

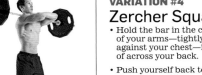

VARIATION #3
Crossed-Arm Barbell Front Squat

- Set a bar on a squat rack and cross your arms in front of you so that each hand is on top of the bar.

- Step under the bar so that it's resting on the tops of your shoulders, and raise your arms so that the bar can't roll off them.

- Step back and perform a squat, keeping your arms in the same position for the entire movement.

- Push yourself back to a standing position.

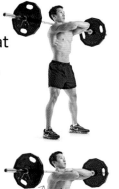

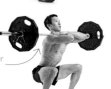

Don't let your arms drop.

VARIATION #4
Zercher Squat

- Hold the bar in the crooks of your arms—tightly against your chest—instead of across your back.

- Push yourself back to a standing position.

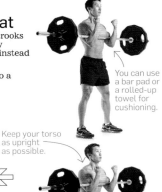

You can use a bar pad or a rolled-up towel for cushioning.

Keep your torso as upright as possible.

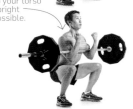

The Zercher squat not only strengthens your lower body but also works your biceps and front deltoids, muscles that have to stay contracted in order to hold the bar.

VARIATION #5
Barbell Siff Squat

- Before you squat, raise your heels as high as you can and hold them that way for the entire lift.

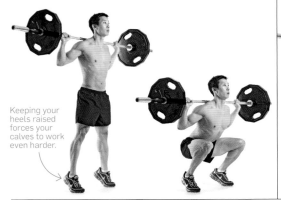

Keeping your heels raised forces your calves to work even harder.

VARIATION #6
Barbell Quarter Squat

- Lower your body only until your knees are bent about 60 degrees.

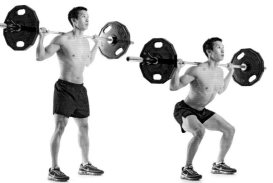

MAIN MOVE
Dumbbell Squat

A

- Hold a pair of dumbbells at arm's length next to your sides, your palms facing each other.

B

- Brace your abs, and lower your body as far as you can by pushing your hips back and bending your knees.
- Pause, then slowly push yourself back to the starting position.

KEEP YOUR HEAD UP
Looking down when you squat puts you at greater risk of injury, say scientists at Miami University of Ohio. The researchers found that gazing down during the movement causes your body to lean forward 4 to 5 degrees. This increases the strain on your lower back. Looking at yourself in the mirror can also cause a forward lean. Your best approach: Before you descend, find a mark that's stable and just above eye level, and stay focused on it throughout the movement.

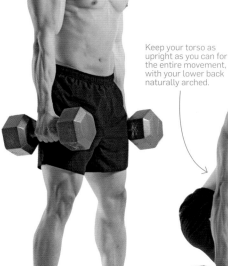

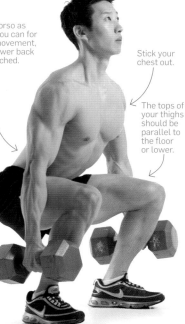

Keep your torso as upright as you can for the entire movement, with your lower back naturally arched.

Stick your chest out.

The tops of your thighs should be parallel to the floor or lower.

Keep your weight on your heels, not on your toes, for the entire movement.

103

Quads & Calves | SQUATS

VARIATION #1
Goblet Squat

- Hold a dumbbell vertically next to your chest, with both hands cupping the dumbbell head. (Imagine that it's a heavy goblet.)

- Pause, then push yourself back to the starting position.

Don't be afraid to lower your body as deep as possible. Research shows that the most unstable knee angle during the squat is when your knees are bent 90 degrees—a few inches above the point where your upper thighs are parallel to the floor.

Your elbows should brush the insides of your knees; in fact, it's perfectly fine if they push your knees outward.

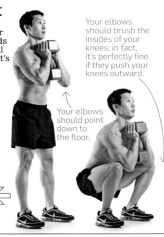

Your elbows should point down to the floor.

VARIATION #2
Wide-Stance Goblet Squat

- With both hands, hold a dumbbell vertically next to your chest.

Keep your torso as upright as possible.

Set your feet about twice shoulder-width apart, your toes pointing out at an angle.

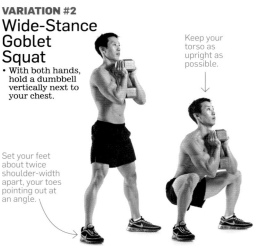

VARIATION #3
Sumo Squat

- Grasp a head of a heavy dumbbell in each hand, and hold the weight at arm's length in front of your waist.

Keep your lower back naturally arched for the entire movement.

Set your feet at about twice shoulder width, your toes turned out slightly.

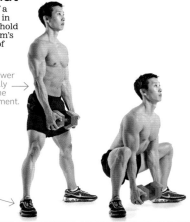

VARIATION #4
Dumbbell Front Squat

- Hold a pair of dumbbells so that your palms are facing each other, and rest one of the dumbbell heads on the meatiest part of each shoulder.

- Keep your body as upright as you can at all times.

- Don't allow your elbows to drop down as you squat.

Keeping your upper arms parallel to the floor helps to keep your torso from leaning forward excessively.

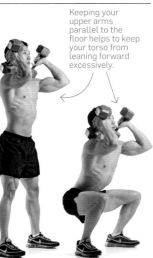

VARIATION #5
Dumbbell Jump Squat

A

- Hold a pair of dumbbells at arm's length next to your sides, your palms facing each other.
- Dip your knees in preparation to leap.

> **JUMP HIGHER, RUN FASTER**
> *You can boost your vertical and improve your speed with a simple jump squat routine, according to an 8-week study in the Journal of Strength and Conditioning. In the study, subjects used a weight that was 30 percent of the amount they could squat one time. Try it yourself: Twice a week, do five sets of six reps, resting 3 minutes after each set.*

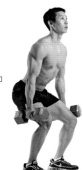

B

- Explosively jump as high as you can.
- When you land, reset quickly before jumping again.

Land as softly as you can on the balls of your feet, then lower your heels back to the floor.

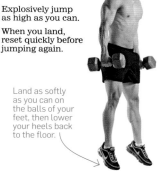

VARIATION #6
Overhead Dumbbell Squat

A

- Hold a pair of dumbbells straight over your shoulders, your arms completely straight.

43

Percent reduction in knee pain after sufferers performed lower body exercises such as the squat for 4 months, according to a Tufts University study.

B

- Lower your body until your upper thighs are at least parallel to the floor.

Brace your core.

Set your feet slightly wider than hip-width apart.

Your lower back should stay naturally arched for the entire movement.

Don't let the dumbbells fall forward as you squat.

Keep your torso as upright as possible.

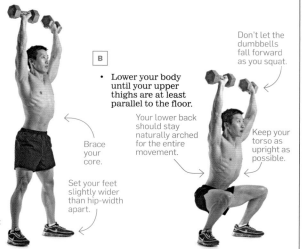

MUSCLE MISTAKE
You Think Smith Machine Squats Are Superior

While the Smith machine—a squat rack with a bar that runs on guides—may look like a foolproof way to squat, it has a major flaw. The bar must travel straight up and down instead of in an arc as it does in a barbell squat. This places more stress on your lower back. What's more, Canadian scientists found that free-weight squats activate the quads almost 50 percent more than Smith machine squats.

Quads & Calves | SQUATS

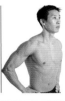

MAIN MOVE
Dumbbell Split Squat

TRAINER'S TIP
Try the Barbell Split Squat. Hold a bar across your upper back with an overhand grip.

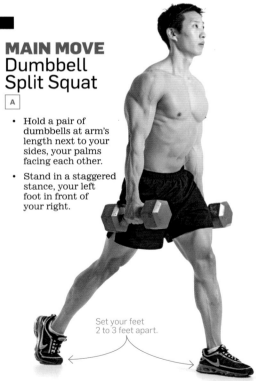

A

- Hold a pair of dumbbells at arm's length next to your sides, your palms facing each other.

- Stand in a staggered stance, your left foot in front of your right.

B

- Slowly lower your body as far as you can.

- Pause, then push yourself back up to the starting position as quickly as you can.

- Complete the prescribed number of reps with your left foot forward, then do the same number with your right foot in front of your left.

Set your feet 2 to 3 feet apart.

Keep your torso upright and brace your core for the entire movement.

Your rear knee should nearly touch the floor.

VARIATION #1
Elevated-Front-Foot Dumbbell Split Squat
- Place your front foot on a 6-inch step or box.

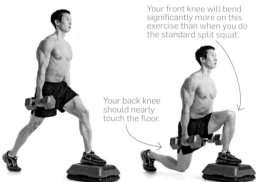

Your front knee will bend significantly more on this exercise than when you do the standard split squat.

Your back knee should nearly touch the floor.

VARIATION #2
Elevated-Back-Foot Dumbbell Split Squat
- Place your back foot on a 6-inch step or box.

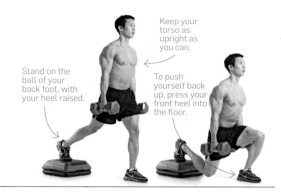

Keep your torso as upright as you can.

Stand on the ball of your back foot, with your heel raised.

To push yourself back up, press your front heel into the floor.

VARIATION #3
Overhead Dumbbell Split Squat
- Hold a pair of dumbbells directly over your shoulders, with your arms completely straight.

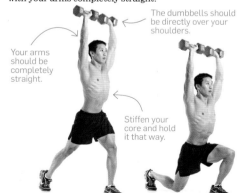

The dumbbells should be directly over your shoulders.

Your arms should be completely straight.

Stiffen your core and hold it that way.

VARIATION #4
Dumbbell Bulgarian Split Squat
- Place just the instep of your back foot on a bench.

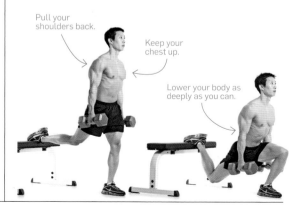

Pull your shoulders back.

Keep your chest up.

Lower your body as deeply as you can.

Quads & Calves | LUNGES

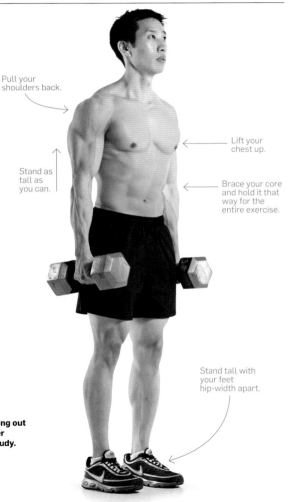

Pull your
shoulders back.

Lift your
chest up.

Stand as
tall as
you can.

Brace your core
and hold it that
way for the
entire exercise.

MAIN MOVE
Dumbbell Lunge

A

- Grab a pair of dumbbells and hold them at arm's length next to your sides, your palms facing each other.

Stand tall with
your feet
hip-width apart.

50

**Percent less likely people were to die
of heart disease when they first started working out
in their 40s compared to those who never
got off the couch, according to a German study.**

BODY-WEIGHT LUNGE
You can do just about any version of the lunge without holding weights of any kind. Simply cross your arms in front of your chest, or place your hands on your hips or behind your ears. These are ideal warmup exercises and are also valuable as great alternatives to the weighted variations.

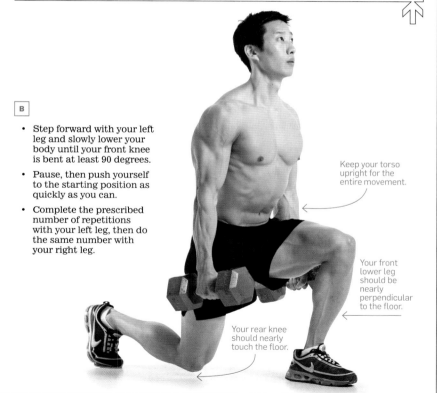

B

- Step forward with your left leg and slowly lower your body until your front knee is bent at least 90 degrees.

- Pause, then push yourself to the starting position as quickly as you can.

- Complete the prescribed number of repetitions with your left leg, then do the same number with your right leg.

Keep your torso upright for the entire movement.

Your front lower leg should be nearly perpendicular to the floor.

Your rear knee should nearly touch the floor.

VARIATION #1
Alternating Dumbbell Lunge
- Instead of performing all of your reps with one leg before repeating with the other, alternate back and forth—doing one rep with your left, then one rep with your right.

VARIATION #2
Walking Dumbbell Lunge
- Instead of pushing your body backward to the starting position, raise up and bring your back foot forward so that you move forward (like you're walking) a step with every rep. Alternate the leg you step forward with each time.

VARIATION #3
Reverse Dumbbell Lunge
- Step backward with your right leg. Then lower your body into a lunge. This looks the same in a photo as the dumbbell lunge. Do all your reps and repeat with your other leg. You can also use the alternating technique.

109

Quads & Calves | LUNGES

VARIATION #4
Dumbbell Box Lunge
- Place a 6-inch step or box about 2 feet in front of you.
- Step forward onto the box with your left leg, and then lower your body into a lunge.

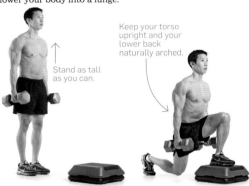

Stand as tall as you can.

Keep your torso upright and your lower back naturally arched.

VARIATION #5
Reverse Dumbbell Box Lunge
- Stand on a 6-inch step or box, and step backward with your left leg into a lunge.

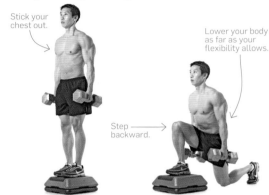

Stick your chest out.

Lower your body as far as your flexibility allows.

Step backward.

VARIATION #6
Dumbbell Stepover

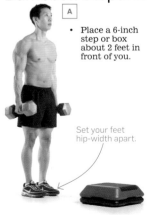

A
- Place a 6-inch step or box about 2 feet in front of you.

Set your feet hip-width apart.

B
- Step forward onto the step with your left foot as you lower your body into a lunge.

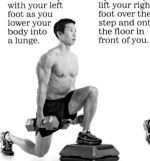

C
- Push yourself up so that you lift your right foot over the step and onto the floor in front of you.

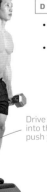

D
- Lower yourself into a lunge.
- Reverse the movement to return to the starting position.

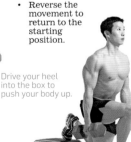

Drive your heel into the box to push your body up.

VARIATION #7
Reverse Dumbbell Box Lunge with Forward Reach

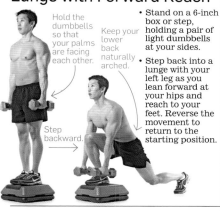

Hold the dumbbells so that your palms are facing each other.

Keep your lower back naturally arched.

Step backward.

- Stand on a 6-inch box or step, holding a pair of light dumbbells at your sides.
- Step back into a lunge with your left leg as you lean forward at your hips and reach to your feet. Reverse the movement to return to the starting position.

VARIATION #8
Dumbbell Crossover Lunge
- Instead of stepping directly forward when you lunge, cross your lead foot in front of your back foot, as if you were doing a curtsy.

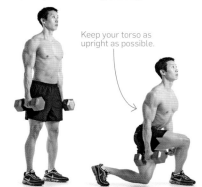

Keep your torso as upright as possible.

VARIATION #9
Reverse Dumbbell Crossover Lunge
- Instead of stepping forward, step backward and cross your rear foot behind your front foot.

VARIATION #10
Dumbbell Lunge and Rotation

If you're stepping forward with your left leg, rotate your torso to your left side. If you're stepping with your right, rotate to your right.

- Grab a dumbbell and hold it by the ends, just below your chin.
- Step forward into a lunge. As you lunge, rotate your upper body toward the same side as the leg you're using to step forward.

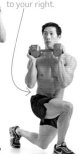

Brace your core and hold it that way for the entire movement.

VARIATION #11
Overhead Dumbbell Lunge
- Hold a pair of dumbbells directly over your shoulders, with your arms completely straight.
- Step forward with your left leg into a lunge.

Don't allow the weight to carry you forward. Instead, think about dropping your hips straight down as you step forward. Keep your abs tight and your chest up.

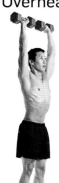

VARIATION #12
Overhead Dumbbell Reverse Lunge
- This time, step backward with your right leg into a lunge.

Quads & Calves |

VARIATION #13
Offset Dumbbell Lunge

- Hold a dumbbell in your right hand next to your shoulder, with your arm bent.

- Step forward into a lunge with your right foot.

- Complete the prescribed number of reps on that side, then switch arms and lunge with your left leg for the same number of reps.

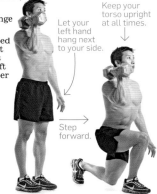

Keep your torso upright at all times.

Let your left hand hang next to your side.

Step forward.

STRENGTHEN YOUR CORE
Holding a weight on just one side of your body increases the demand placed on your core to keep your body stable.

VARIATION #14
Offset Dumbbell Reverse Lunge

- Hold a dumbbell in your left hand next to your shoulder, with your arm bent.

- Step backward into a lunge with your right foot.

- Complete the prescribed number of reps on that side, then switch arms and lunge backward with your left leg for the same number of reps.

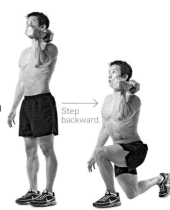

Step backward.

VARIATION #15
Dumbbell Rotational Lunge

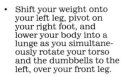 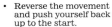

- Hold a pair of dumbbells at arm's length next to your sides, your palms facing each other.

- Lift your left foot and step to the left and back, placing that foot so it's diagonal to your body and pointed toward 8 o'clock.

- Shift your weight onto your left leg, pivot on your right foot, and lower your body into a lunge as you simultaneously rotate your torso and the dumbbells to the left, over your front leg.

- Reverse the movement and push yourself back up to the start.

- Complete the prescribed number of reps with your left leg, then do the same number with your right leg. (Your right foot will point to 4 o'clock.)

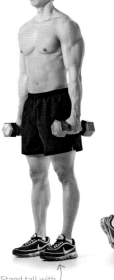

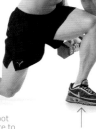

Keep your core braced as you rotate your torso.

Stand tall with your feet hip-width apart, pointing ahead to 12 o'clock.

Your right foot should rotate to point in the same direction as your left foot.

Your left foot should point to 8 o'clock in relation to your starting position.

VARIATION #16
Dumbbell Side Lunge

- Hold a pair of dumbbells at arm's length next to your sides, your palms facing each other.

- Lift your left foot and take a big step to your left as you push your hips backward and lower your body by dropping your hips and bending your left knee.

- Pause, then quickly push yourself back to the starting position.

Your right foot should remain flat on the floor.

Your feet should be pointed straight ahead in both the up and the down positions.

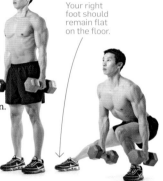

VARIATION #17
Dumbbell Diagonal Lunge

- Instead of stepping straight forward, lunge diagonally at a 45-degree angle.

- Complete all your reps, then switch legs and repeat.

Lunge forward or back in this direction.

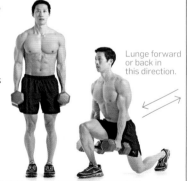

VARIATION #18
Reverse Dumbbell Diagonal Lunge

- You can also perform this exercise by lunging backward at a 45-degree angle.

VARIATION #19
Dumbbell Side Lunge and Touch

If you can't touch the floor without rounding your lower back, only lower as far as you can while keeping your back naturally arched.

You'll have to lean forward at your hips, but focus on keeping your head and chest up, instead of allowing your torso to slump forward.

Don't allow your right foot to raise up off the floor.

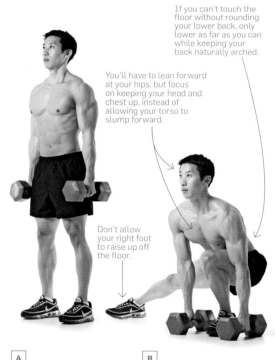

A
- Hold a pair of dumbbells at arm's length next to your sides.

B
- As you lower your body into a side lunge, bend forward at your hips and touch the dumbbells to the floor.

113

Quads & Calves | CALF RAISES

CALF RAISES
The targets for these exercises are your gastrocnemius and soleus muscles.

MAIN MOVE
Standing Barbell Calf Raise

A

- Grab a barbell with an overhand grip and place it so that it rests comfortably across your upper back.
- Place the ball of each foot on a 25-pound weight plate.

B

- Rise up on your toes as high as you can.
- Pause, then slowly lower back to the starting position.

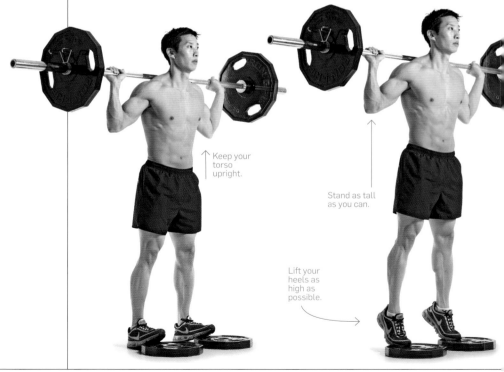

Keep your torso upright.

Stand as tall as you can.

Lift your heels as high as possible.

114

VARIATION #1

Single-Leg Standing Dumbbell Calf Raise

A

- Grab a dumbbell in your right hand and stand on a step, block, or 25-pound weight plate.
- Cross your left foot behind your right ankle, and balance yourself on the ball of your right foot, with your right heel onthe floor or hanging off a step.

Put your left hand on something stable—a wall or weight stack, for instance.

B

- Lift your right heel as high as you can. Pause, then lower and repeat.
- Complete the prescribed number of reps with your right leg, then do the same number with your left (while holding the dumbbell in your left hand).

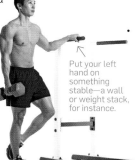
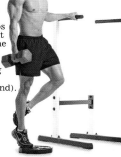

VARIATION #2

Single-Leg Bent-Knee Calf Raise

- Bend your knee, and hold it that way as you perform the exercise.

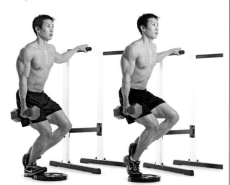

VARIATION #3

Single-Leg Donkey Calf Raise

- Keeping your back naturally arched, bend at your hips and lower your torso until your upper body is almost parallel to the floor.
- Complete the prescribed number of reps with your right leg, then do the same number with your left.

Don't round your lower back.

Place your hands on a sturdy object for support.

Raise your heel as high as you can.

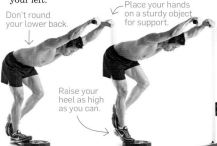

Bend for More Muscle

Of the two muscles that make up your calf, your soleus is more involved in extending your ankle when your knee is bent. Your gastrocnemius takes on a greater work-load when your knee is straight. As a result, bent-leg calf raises target your soleus best, while standing calf raises—performed with your knee straight—zero in on your gastrocnemius. That's why if your calves don't seem to be growing, many experts recommend doing both versions of the exercise.

115

Quads & Calves

THE BEST QUADRICEPS EXERCISE YOU'VE NEVER DONE
Wide-Grip Overhead Barbell Split Squat

This movement is known as a "big bang" exercise since it works so many muscles at once. While your legs are the obvious emphasis during the split-squat portion of the move, holding the weight over your head challenges your shoulders, arms, upper back, and core, too. So it's a great strength and muscle builder, but it also burns tons of calories. If you're intimidated by holding a barbell overhead, start by performing it with just a broomstick or a pole, instead.

A

- Hold a barbell straight over your head with an overhand grip that's about twice shoulder width.
- Stand in a staggered stance with your feet 2 to 3 feet apart.

B

- Slowly lower your body as far as you can.
- Pause, then push yourself back up to the starting position as quickly as you can.
- Complete the prescribed number of repetitions with your left leg forward, then do the same number with your right leg in front.

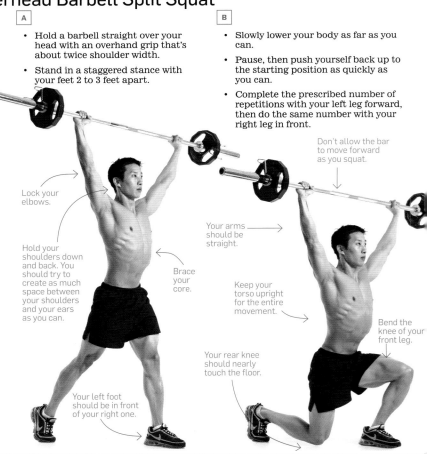

Lock your elbows.

Hold your shoulders down and back. You should try to create as much space between your shoulders and your ears as you can.

Brace your core.

Your left foot should be in front of your right one.

Don't allow the bar to move forward as you squat.

Your arms should be straight.

Keep your torso upright for the entire movement.

Bend the knee of your front leg.

Your rear knee should nearly touch the floor.

■

THE BEST CALF EXERCISE YOU'VE NEVER DONE
Farmer's Walk on Toes

This exercise not only works your calves but also improves your cardiovascular fitness. Choose the heaviest pair of dumbbells that allows you to perform the exercise for 60 seconds. If you feel like you could have gone longer, grab heavier weights on your next set.

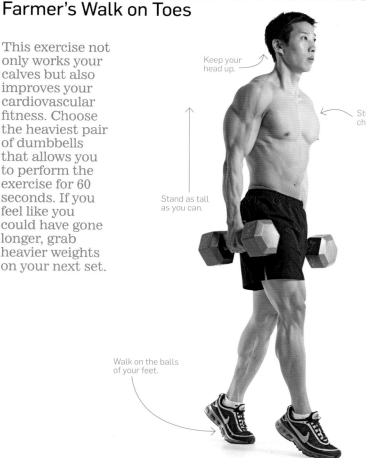

Keep your head up.

Stick your chest out.

Stand as tall as you can.

Walk on the balls of your feet.

A
- Grab a pair of heavy dumbbells and hold them at your sides at arm's length.

B
- Raise your heels and walk forward (or in a circle) for 60 seconds.

Glutes
& Hamstrings

A nytime you're standing, the muscles of your glutes and hamstrings are working. Trouble is, most of us are spending more and more of our days sitting—whether in front of a computer or 46-inch plasma. The impact of so much chair time: Our hip muscles not only become weak, they forget how to contract. This is especially true for your glutes. And that's a shame, since your glutes are your body's largest and perhaps most powerful muscle group.

What's more, when either your glutes or hamstrings are weak, it disrupts the muscular balance of your body, which can cause pain and injuries in your knees, hips, and lower back. The solution? Make working your glutes and hamstrings a top priority, using the exercises in this chapter.

Bonus Benefits

Greater calorie burn! Since the glutes are your biggest muscle group, they're also one of your top calorie burners.

Better posture! Weak glutes can cause your hips to tilt forward. This puts more stress on your spine. It also pushes your lower abdomen outward, making your belly stick out.

Healthier knees! Your anterior cruciate ligaments (ACLs) rely on your hamstrings to help them stabilize your knees. Having a strong set of hamstrings can help your ACLs do their job and lower your risk of injury.

Meet Your Muscles

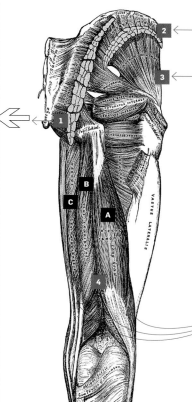

Gluteus Medius and Gluteus Minimus

You have two other glute muscles: your gluteus medius [2] and gluteus minimus [3]. These assist your gluteus maximus in raising your thigh out to the side. They also rotate your thigh outward when your leg is straight and inward when your hip is bent.

Hamstrings

The muscles known collectively as your hamstring [4] are actually three separate muscles: the biceps femoris [A], semitendinosus [B], and semimembranosus [C]. Their primary functions are to bend your knee and to help your gluteus maximus extend your hip. The biceps femoris also helps rotate your thigh outward; the semimembranosus and semitendinosus help rotate it inward.

Gluteus Maximus

You could just call the gluteus maximus [1] your butt muscle. That's because it creates the shape of your rear end. It's working anytime you raise your thigh out to your side, rotate your leg so that your foot is pointing outward, or thrust your hips forward. So if you're in a sitting or squatting position, your gluteus maximus helps you stand up by straightening your hips. As a result, it's working in most lower-body exercises, but particularly during the deadlift, hip raise, and reverse hip raise.

Did You Know?

The tendons of a pig's hamstring muscle can be used to suspend a ham during curing, which explains the origin of the muscle's name.

MUSCLE MISTAKE

You Work Your Quads Harder Than Your Hamstrings

A study in the *American Journal of Sports Medicine* found that 70 percent of athletes with recurrent hamstring injuries suffered from muscle imbalances between their quadriceps and hamstrings. After correcting the imbalances by strengthening the hamstrings, every person in the study went injury-free for the entire 12-month follow-up. Now that's strong medicine.

119

Glutes & Hams |

In this chapter, you'll find 43 exercises that target the muscles of your glutes and hamstrings. Throughout, you'll notice that certain exercises have been given the designation Main Move. Master this basic version of a movement, and you'll be able to do all of its variations with flawless form.

HIP RAISES

These exercises target the muscles of your glutes and hamstrings. What's more, they require you to activate your abdominal and lower-back muscles in order to keep your body stable—so they double as great core exercises.

MAIN MOVE
Hip Raises

A

- Lie faceup on the floor with your knees bent and your feet flat on the floor.

Make sure you're pushing with your heels. To make it easier, you can position your feet so that your toes rise off the floor.

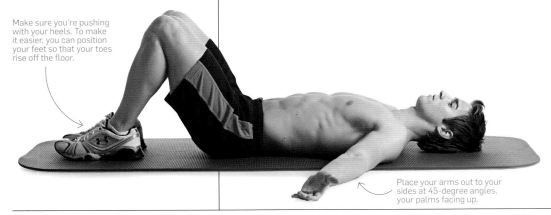

Place your arms out to your sides at 45-degree angles, your palms facing up.

GET YOUR BUTT IN GEAR
If your hamstrings cramp when you perform the hip raise, it's often a sign that your glutes are weak. That's because your hamstrings are having to work extra hard to keep your hips raised. For best results, raise your hips and hold them that way for 3 to 5 seconds per repetition. Twice a week, do two or three sets of 10 to 12 reps.

B

- Raise your hips so your body forms a straight line from your shoulders to your knees.
- Pause for up to 5 seconds in the up position, then lower your body back to the starting position.

15

Minutes of exercise it takes to improve your mood, according to a study in the *Journal of Sports and Exercise Psychology*.

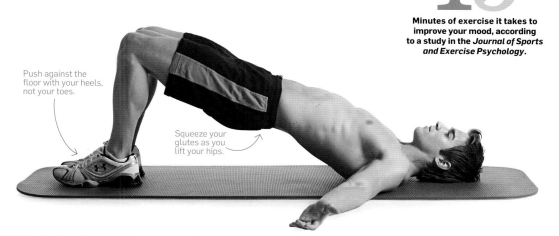

Push against the floor with your heels, not your toes.

Squeeze your glutes as you lift your hips.

Glutes & Hams | HIP RAISES

VARIATION #1
Weighted Hip Raise
• Place a weight plate on your hips and perform the exercise.

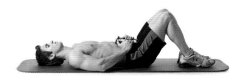

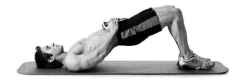

VARIATION #2
Hip Raise with Knee Press-Out
• Place a 20-inch mini-band just above your knees, and keep your knees from touching each other as you perform the movement.

Pushing outward against a band increases the activation of your gluteus maximus and gluteus medius.

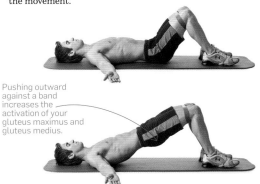

VARIATION #3
Hip Raise with Knee Squeeze

 A

• Place a rolled-up towel or an Airex pad between your knees, and hold it there as you perform the movement.

 B

• Don't allow the pad to slip as you raise your hips until your body forms a straight line from your shoulders to your knees.

TRAINER'S TIP
Pay attention as you raise your hips: If your knees tend to fall outward as you do the exercise, you probably have weak hip adductors, or groin muscles. Keeping a towel or cushion from falling to the floor as you do the exercise helps strengthen these inner-thigh muscles.

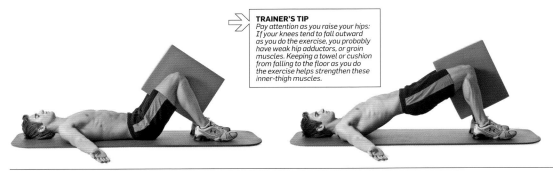

VARIATION #4
Marching Hip Raise

- Raise your hips and hold them that way.

- Lift one knee to your chest, lower back to the start, and lift your other knee to your chest. Continue to alternate back and forth.

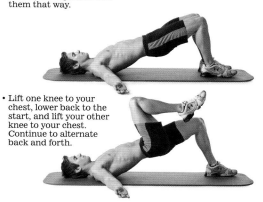

VARIATION #5
Hip Raise with Feet on a Swiss Ball

- Perform the movement with your lower legs placed on a Swiss ball.

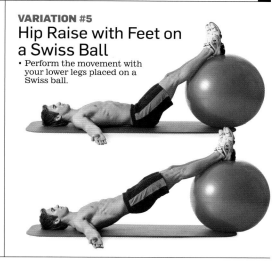

VARIATION #6
Marching Hip Raise with Feet on a Swiss Ball

A

- Place your feet flat on a Swiss ball.

B

- Lift one knee to your chest, lower back to the start, and lift your other knee to your chest. Continue to alternate back and forth.

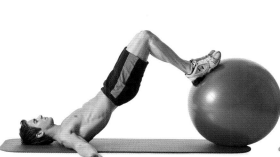

Don't allow your hips to sag.

Glutes & Hams | HIP RAISES

MAIN MOVE
Single-Leg Hip Raise

- Lie faceup on the floor with your left knee bent and your right leg straight.
- Raise your right leg until it's in line with your left thigh.

Place your arms out to your sides at 45-degree angles to your torso, your palms facing up.

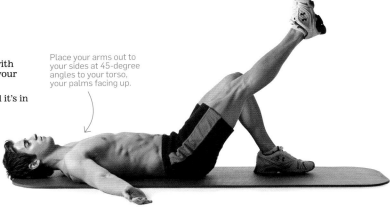

- Push your hips upward, keeping your left leg elevated.
- Pause, then slowly lower your body and leg back to the starting position.
- Complete the prescribed number of repetitions with your left leg, then switch legs and do the same number with your right leg.

Your right leg stays in line with your left thigh when you raise your hips.

Your body should form a straight line from your shoulders to your knees.

You can raise your toes to make sure you're pushing from your heel.

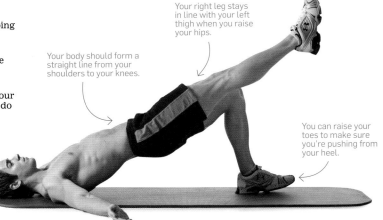

VARIATION #1
Single-Leg Hip Raise with Knee Hold

- Bring one knee toward your chest and hold it there as you perform the exercise.

TRAINER'S TIP
Holding one knee helps ensure you're using your glutes to raise your hips—and not your lower back muscles.

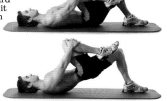

VARIATION #2
Single-Leg Hip Raise with Foot on a Bosu Ball

- Place your left foot on the Bosu ball.
- Raise your hips, lower, and repeat.

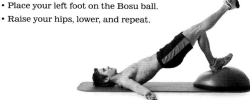

VARIATION #3
Single-Leg Hip Raise with Foot on Step

- Position your butt against a 6-inch step.
- Place your left foot on the step.
- Raise your hips, lower, and repeat.

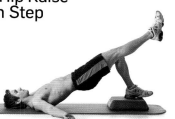

VARIATION #4
Single-Leg Hip Raise with Foot on Bench

- Place your left heel on a bench, with your butt on the floor.
- Raise your hips, lower, and repeat.

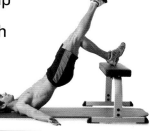

VARIATION #5
Single-Leg Hip Raise with Foot on a Foam Roller

Placing your foot on a foam roller forces your stabilizer muscles to work harder to prevent the roller from moving forward or back.

- Place your left foot on a foam roller.
- Raise your hips, lower, and repeat.

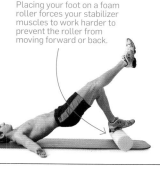

VARIATION #6
Single-Leg Hip Raise with Foot on a Medicine Ball

Placing your foot on a medicine ball forces your stabilizer muscles to work harder to prevent the ball from moving forward or back, or from side to side.

- Place your left foot on a medicine ball.
- Raise your hips, lower, and repeat.

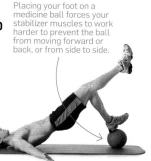

Glutes & Hams |

VARIATION #7
Hip Raise with Head on a Bosu Ball
• Place your head and upper back on a Bosu ball.

Elevating your upper body increases the demand on your glutes.

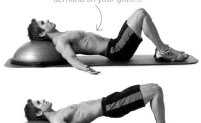

VARIATION #8
Single-Leg Hip Raise with Head on a Bosu Ball
• Place your head and upper back on a Bosu ball, and hold your right leg in the air so that it's in line with your left thigh.

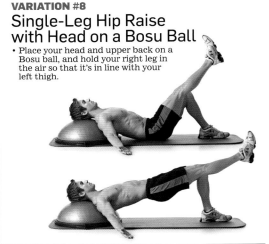

VARIATION #9
Hip Raise with Head on a Swiss Ball
• Place your head and upper back on a Swiss ball.

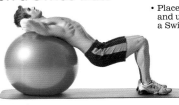

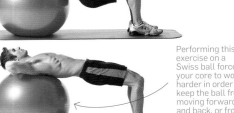

Performing this exercise on a Swiss ball forces your core to work harder in order to keep the ball from moving forward and back, or from side to side.

VARIATION #10
Single-Leg Hip Raise with Head on a Swiss Ball
• Place your head and upper back on a Swiss ball, and lift your right leg in the air so that it's in line with your left thigh.

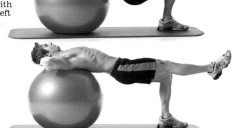

MAIN MOVE
Swiss-Ball Hip Raise and Leg Curl

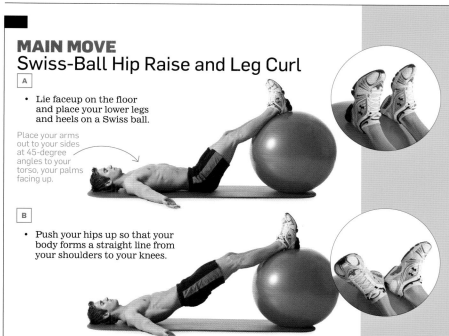

A

- Lie faceup on the floor and place your lower legs and heels on a Swiss ball.

Place your arms out to your sides at 45-degree angles to your torso, your palms facing up.

B

- Push your hips up so that your body forms a straight line from your shoulders to your knees.

C

- Without pausing, pull your heels toward you and roll the ball as close as possible to your butt.

- Pause for 1 or 2 seconds, then reverse the motion by rolling the ball back until your body is in a straight line. Lower your hips back to the floor.

Focus on keeping your hips in line with the rest of your body as you pull the ball toward you.

Muscle Moves

When doing the standard Swiss-ball hip raise and leg curl, your feet should point up. But by turning them in or out, you can change the part of your hamstrings that is targeted.

VARIATION #1
Swiss-Ball Hip Raise and Leg Curl with Toes Out
Place your lower legs on the ball with your heels touching and your toes pointing outward.

Turning your feet out emphasizes the hamstring muscles on the outside portion of your leg.

VARIATION #2
Swiss-Ball Hip Raise and Leg Curl with Toes In
Place your lower legs on the ball with your heels about shoulder-width apart and your toes pointing toward each other.

Turning your feet in emphasizes the hamstring muscles on the inside portion of your leg.

Glutes & Hams | HIP RAISES

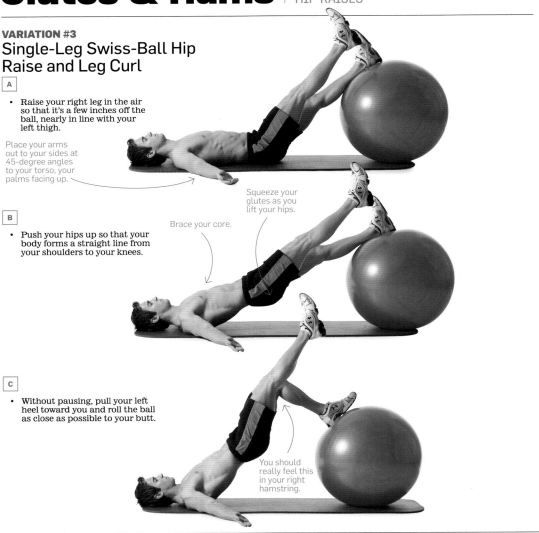

VARIATION #3
Single-Leg Swiss-Ball Hip Raise and Leg Curl

A

- Raise your right leg in the air so that it's a few inches off the ball, nearly in line with your left thigh.

Place your arms out to your sides at 45-degree angles to your torso, your palms facing up.

Squeeze your glutes as you lift your hips.

Brace your core.

B

- Push your hips up so that your body forms a straight line from your shoulders to your knees.

C

- Without pausing, pull your left heel toward you and roll the ball as close as possible to your butt.

You should really feel this in your right hamstring.

MAIN MOVE
Sliding Leg Curl

- Lie faceup on the floor and place each heel on a Valslide with your knees bent and your heels near your butt.

Brace your core and squeeze your glutes as you lift your hips.

- Keeping your hips in line with your torso, slide your heels out until your legs are straight.

- Reverse the movement back to the starting position.

Your body should form a straight line from your shoulders to your knees.

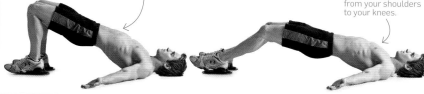

VARIATION
Single-Leg Sliding Leg Curl

A

- Raise your left leg in the air so that it's in line with your right thigh, and hold it that way as you perform the exercise.

B

- Keeping your hips in line with your torso, slide your heel out until your leg is straight.

Your body should form a straight line from your shoulders to your knees.

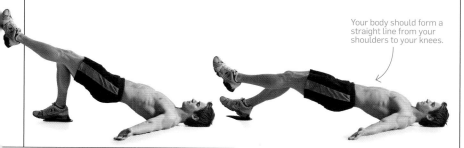

MUSCLE MISTAKE
You Only Do Machine Leg Curls

The machine leg curl requires you to flex your knees, a movement that is one of the jobs of your hamstrings. However, the main function of your hamstrings is to extend or push your hips forward, as you do in straight-leg deadlifts and hip raises. What's more, another type of leg curl—the Swiss-ball hip raise and leg curl—requires both knee flexion and hip extension. So it's a better choice than the classic machine version, too.

Glutes & Hams | BENT-KNEE DEADLIFTS

BENT-KNEE DEADLIFTS

These exercises target the muscles of your glutes and hamstrings, along with scores of others. In fact, because deadlifts strongly activate your quadriceps, core, back, and shoulder muscles, too, they're among the best total-body exercises you can do.

MAIN MOVE
Barbell Deadlift

- Load the barbell and roll it against your shins.
- Bend at your hips and knees and grab the bar with an overhand grip, your hands just beyond shoulder width.

- Without allowing your lower back to round, pull your torso back and up, thrust your hips forward, and stand up with the barbell.
- Squeeze your glutes as you perform the movement.
- Lower the bar to the floor, keeping it as close to your body as possible.

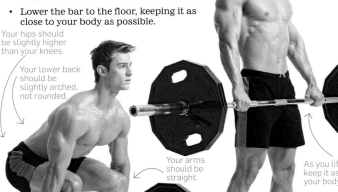

Your hips should be slightly higher than your knees.

Your lower back should be slightly arched, not rounded.

Your arms should be straight.

As you lift the bar, keep it as close to your body as possible.

TRAINER'S TIP
You can also perform the deadlift and wide-grip deadlift while standing with each foot on a 25-pound weight plate. This increases the distance you have to lift the weight, challenging your muscles even more.

VARIATION #1
Wide-Grip Barbell Deadlift

A

- Use an overhand grip that's about twice shoulder width.

B

- Once standing, reverse the movement and slowly lower the bar back to the floor.

THE ULTIMATE DEADLIFT?
Using a wider grip provides three bonus benefits: (1) It increases the demand on your upper-back muscles, (2) forces your forearm and hand muscles to work harder, and (3) boosts your range of motion.

This exercise is also called a snatch-grip deadlift, since you grasp the bar with the same grip that Olympic weightlifters use when performing the snatch.

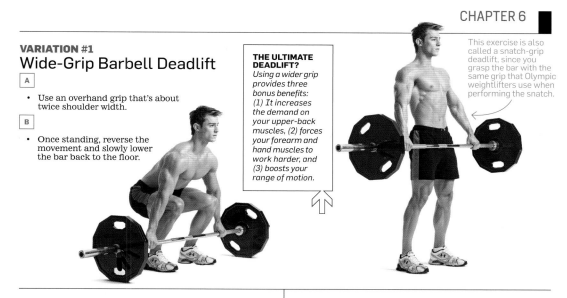

VARIATION #2
Single-Leg Barbell Deadlift

- Place the instep of one foot on a bench that's about 2 feet behind you.

- Complete the prescribed number of reps with your right foot on the bench, then do the same number with your left foot on the bench.

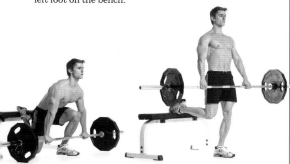

VARIATION #3
Sumo Deadlift

- Stand with your feet about twice shoulder-width apart and your toes pointed out at an angle.

- Grasp the center of the bar with your hands 12 inches apart and palms facing you.

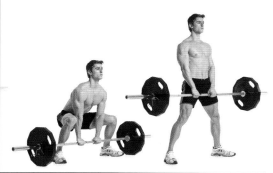

Glutes & Hams | BENT-KNEE DEADLIFTS

MAIN MOVE
Dumbbell Deadlift

A

- Set a pair of dumbbells on the floor in front of you.
- Bend at your hips and knees, and grab the dumbbells with an overhand grip.

B

- Without allowing your lower back to round, stand up with the dumbbells.
- Lower the dumbbells to the floor. (If you can't lower the dumbbells all the way to the floor while keeping a slight arch in your lower back, stop just above the point where it starts to round.)

1,008

Most weight, in pounds, ever deadlifted in competition.

Your arms should be straight, and your lower back slightly arched, not rounded.

As you rise, pull your torso back and up.

Thrust your hips forward.

Keep your chest up.

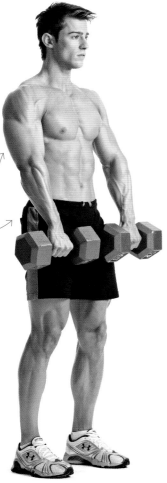

132

VARIATION #1
Single-Arm Deadlift

A

- Use just one dumbbell for this version of the exercise. Place the dumbbell on the floor next to your right ankle. If you can't pick up the dumbbell while keeping a slight arch in your lower back, start the exercise just above the point where your lower back starts to round. (As shown in the photo.)

B

- Complete the prescribed number of repetitions with the weight in your right hand, then do the same number with it in your left.

> This exercise is also called the suitcase deadlift, since it's the same movement you use to pick up luggage.

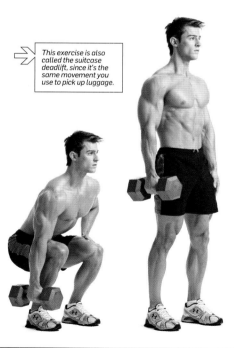

VARIATION #2
Single-Leg Dumbbell Deadlift

A

- Grab a pair of light dumbbells and stand on your left foot.
- Lift your right foot behind you and bend your knee so your right lower leg is parallel to the floor.

B

- Bend forward at your hips, and slowly lower your body as far as you can, or until your right lower leg almost touches the floor.
- Pause, then push your body back to the starting position.
- Complete the prescribed number of reps while standing on your left leg, then do the same number on your right leg.

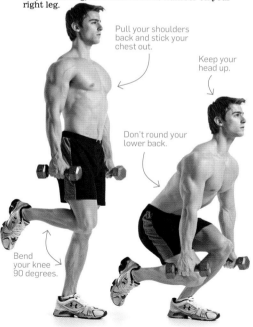

Pull your shoulders back and stick your chest out.

Keep your head up.

Don't round your lower back.

Bend your knee 90 degrees.

Glutes & Hams |

STRAIGHT-LEG DEADLIFTS

These exercises target the muscles of your glutes and hamstrings. They also work your core, especially the muscles of your lower back. One other benefit: They can help improve the flexibility of your hamstrings, since they stretch those muscles every time you lower the weight.

MAIN MOVE
Barbell Straight-Leg Deadlift

A

- Grab a barbell with an overhand grip that's just beyond shoulder width, and hold it at arm's length in front of your hips.

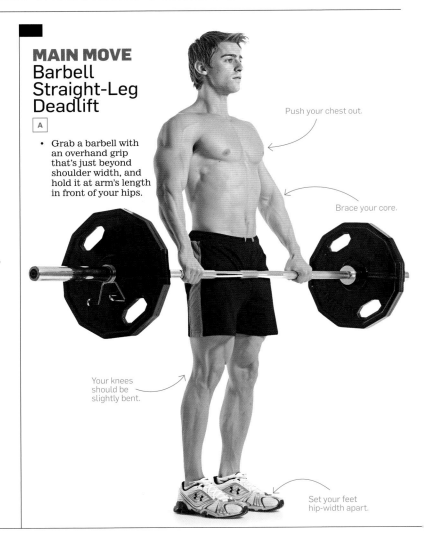

Push your chest out.

Brace your core.

Your knees should be slightly bent.

Set your feet hip-width apart.

TRAINER'S TIP
To lift your torso back to the starting position, squeeze your glutes and thrust your hips forward. This ensures you're engaging your hip muscles, instead of relying more on your lower back.

B

- Without changing the bend in your knees, bend at your hips and lower your torso until it's almost parallel to the floor.

- Pause, then raise your torso back to the starting position.

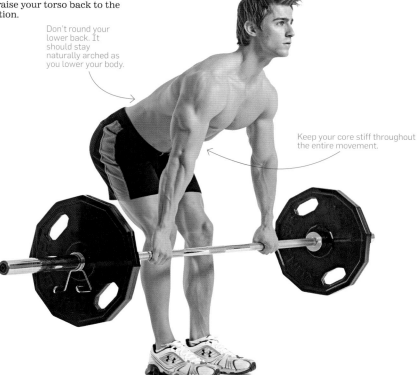

Don't round your lower back. It should stay naturally arched as you lower your body.

Keep your core stiff throughout the entire movement.

Glutes & Hams |

VARIATION #1
Single-Leg Barbell Straight-Leg Deadlift

- Perform the movement while balanced on one leg, instead of two.
- Complete the prescribed number of repetitions with the same leg, then do the same number on your other leg.

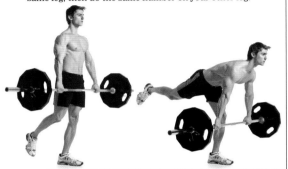

VARIATION #2
Barbell Good Morning

- Instead of holding the barbell at arm's length in front of your body, position it across your upper back and hold it with an overhand grip.

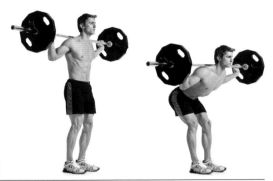

VARIATION #3
Split Barbell Good Morning

A

- Position the barbell across your upper back and hold it with an overhand grip.
- Stand about a foot in front of a 6-inch step, and place your left heel on it.

B

- Keeping your lower back naturally arched, bend forward at your hips as far as you comfortably can.
- Pause, then raise your torso back to the starting position.

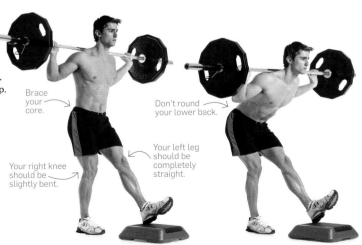

Brace your core.

Don't round your lower back.

Your right knee should be slightly bent.

Your left leg should be completely straight.

MAIN MOVE
Dumbbell Straight-Leg Deadlift

A

- Grab a pair of dumbbells with an overhand grip, and hold them at arm's length in front of your thighs.
- Stand with your feet hip-width apart and your knees slightly bent.

B

- Without changing the bend in your knees, bend at your hips, and lower your torso until it's almost parallel to the floor.
- Pause, then raise your torso back to the starting position.

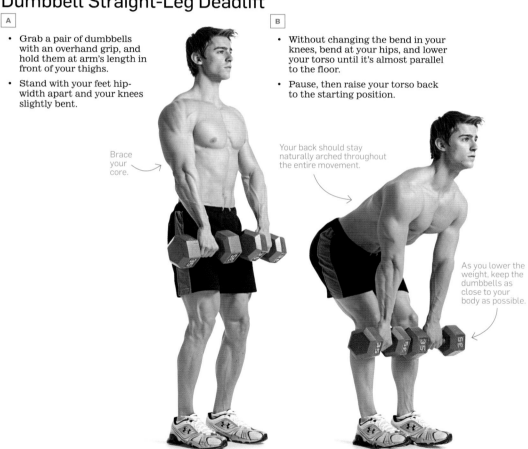

Brace your core.

Your back should stay naturally arched throughout the entire movement.

As you lower the weight, keep the dumbbells as close to your body as possible.

Glutes & Hams |

VARIATION #1
Single-Leg Dumbbell Straight-Leg Deadlift

- Perform a dumbbell straight-leg deadlift while balanced on one leg, instead of two.

- Complete the prescribed number of repetitions with the same leg, then do the same number on your other leg.

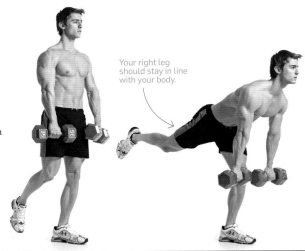

Your right leg should stay in line with your body.

VARIATION #2
Rotational Dumbbell Straight-Leg Deadlift

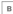

- Grab a light dumbbell in your right hand and stand on your left foot with your knee slightly bent.
- Lift your right foot off the floor and bend your knee slightly.

- Without changing the bend in your left knee, bend at your hips and lower your torso as you rotate it to the left and touch the dumbbell to your left foot.
- Pause, then raise your torso back to the starting position.
- Complete the prescribed number of repetitions standing on your left foot, with the weight in your right hand. Then do the same number on your right foot, with the weight in your left hand.

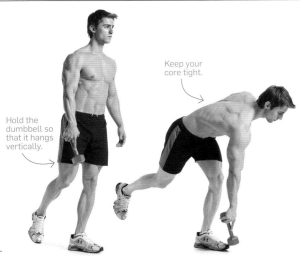

Hold the dumbbell so that it hangs vertically.

Keep your core tight.

MAIN MOVE
Cable Pull Through

A

- Attach a rope handle to the low pulley of a cable machine.
- Grab an end of the rope in each hand and stand with your back to the weight stack.
- Bend at your hips and knees and lower your torso until it's at about a 45-degree angle to the floor.

B

- Thrust your hips forward and raise your torso back to the starting position.

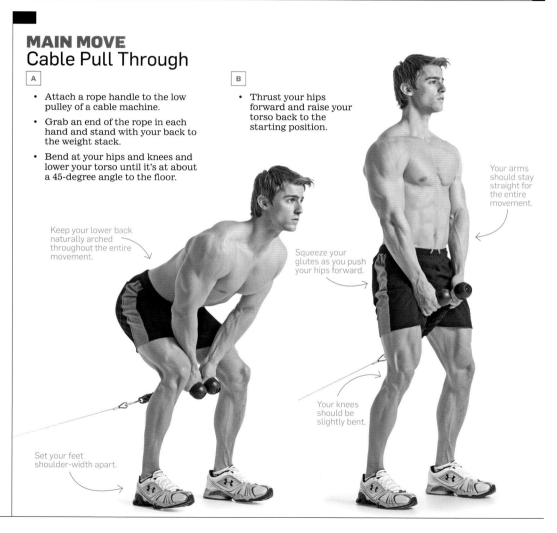

Your arms should stay straight for the entire movement.

Keep your lower back naturally arched throughout the entire movement.

Squeeze your glutes as you push your hips forward.

Your knees should be slightly bent.

Set your feet shoulder-width apart.

Glutes & Hams | STEPUPS

STEPUPS

These exercises target the muscles of your glutes and hamstrings. That's because you have to push your hips forward forcefully to perform the movements. Stepups also work your quadriceps, since they require you to straighten your knee against resistance.

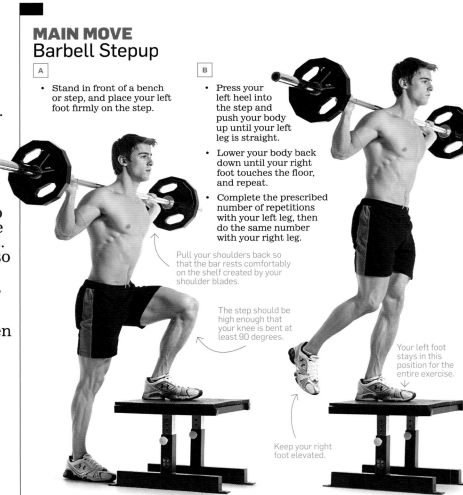

MAIN MOVE
Barbell Stepup

A

- Stand in front of a bench or step, and place your left foot firmly on the step.

B

- Press your left heel into the step and push your body up until your left leg is straight.

- Lower your body back down until your right foot touches the floor, and repeat.

- Complete the prescribed number of repetitions with your left leg, then do the same number with your right leg.

Pull your shoulders back so that the bar rests comfortably on the shelf created by your shoulder blades.

The step should be high enough that your knee is bent at least 90 degrees.

Your left foot stays in this position for the entire exercise.

Keep your right foot elevated.

∎
MAIN MOVE
Dumbbell Stepup

A

- Grab a pair of dumbbells and hold them at arm's length at your sides. Stand in front of a bench or step, and place your left foot firmly on the step.

- The step should be high enough that your knee is bent 90 degrees.

B

- Press your left heel into the step and push your body up until your left leg is straight and you're standing on one leg on the bench, keeping your right foot elevated.

- Lower your body back down until your right foot touches the floor. That's one repetition.

- Complete the prescribed number of repetitions with your left leg, then do the same number with your right leg.

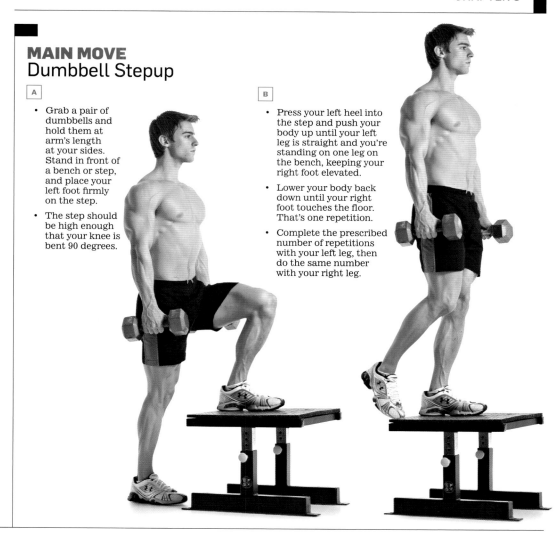

Glutes & Hams | STEPUPS

VARIATION #1
Lateral Dumbbell Stepup

A

- Grab a pair of dumbbells and stand with your left side next to a step.
- Place your left foot on the step.

B

- Press your left foot into the bench and push your body up until both legs are straight.
- Lower back down to the starting position.
- Complete the prescribed number of reps with your left leg, then do the same number with your right leg.

VARIATION #2
Crossover Dumbbell Stepup

A

- Grab a pair of dumbbells and stand with your left side next to a step.
- Place your right foot on the step.

B

- Press your right foot into the bench and push your body up until both legs are straight.
- Lower your body back down to the starting position.
- Complete the prescribed number of reps with your right leg, then do the same number with your left leg.

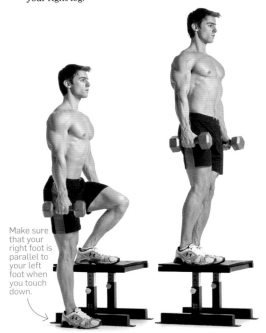

Make sure that your right foot is parallel to your left foot when you touch down.

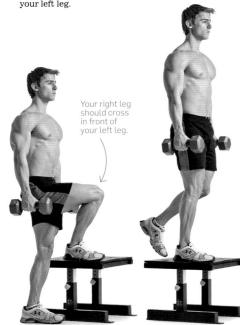

Your right leg should cross in front of your left leg.

THE BEST EXERCISE YOU'VE NEVER DONE
Single-Arm Dumbbell Swing

This movement works your hamstrings and glutes explosively. That means you'll target your very important fast-twitch muscle fibers. These are the fibers that atrophy fastest with age and that are crucial in almost every activity you do—even simply raising yourself out of a chair. So you might say this exercise will help keep your body young. It also works your core, quadriceps, and shoulder muscles, making it a great move for anyone who's short on training time.

A

- Grab a dumbbell with an overhand grip and hold it in front of your waist at arm's length. (You can also do the exercise two handed, holding the dumbbell with both hands.)
- Bend at your hips and knees and lower your torso until it forms a 45-degree angle to the floor.
- Swing the dumbbell between your legs.

B

- Keeping your arm straight, thrust your hips forward, straighten your knees, and swing the dumbbell up to chest level as you rise to standing position.
- Now squat back down as you swing the dumbbell between your legs again.
- Swing the weight back and forth forcefully.

BONUS EXERCISE!
Kettlebell Swing
- Perform the same movement while grasping a kettlebell instead of a dumbbell.

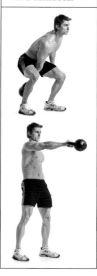

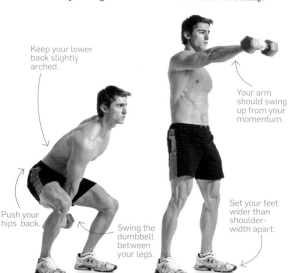

Keep your lower back slightly arched.

Your arm should swing up from your momentum.

Push your hips back.

Swing the dumbbell between your legs.

Set your feet wider than shoulder-width apart.

Core

If the number of infomercial products is any indication, people spend more money on their abs than on any other muscle group. And why wouldn't they? Your abs—or more specifically, your core, which also includes the muscles of your lower back and hips— are involved in every single movement you do. And not just in the gym. If it weren't for your core muscles, you wouldn't even be able to stand or sit upright.

Of course, all of this usually has little to do with most guys' desire for abs that show. Their true motivation is that a visible six-pack is highly appealing to the opposite sex. Perhaps that's because defined abs are an outward sign of a healthy, fit body. The take-home message: Sculpting a rock-solid midsection makes your body not only look better, but work better, too.

Bonus Benefits

Live longer! A Canadian study of more than 8,000 people over 13 years found that those with the weakest abdominal muscles had a death rate more than twice that of the people with the strongest midsections.

Lift more! A stronger core supports your spine, making your entire body more structurally sound. That allows you to use heavier weights on every exercise.

A pain-free back! California State University researchers found that when men followed a 10-week core workout program, they experienced 30 percent less back pain.

Meet Your Muscles

Abdominals

There's no doubt that the most popular abs muscle is the rectus abdominis [1], also known as the six-pack. Despite its nickname, this muscle actually consists of eight segments that are separated by a dense connective tissue called fascia [A]. This muscle is one of those that counteract the pull of the muscles that extend your lower back, helping to keep your spine stable. Its other main duty is to pull your torso toward your hips. That's why you can work this muscle by doing situps and crunches. However, the best way to train your rectus abdominis—and your core as a whole —is with spinal stability exercises, such as the plank and side plank.The abs muscles on the sides of your torso are the external obliques [2] and internal obliques [3]. These muscles help bend your torso to your side, help rotate your torso to your left and right, and perhaps most important, actually act to resist your torso from rotating. So rotational exercises such as the kneeling rotational chop train these muscles, as do antirotation exercises like the kneeling stability chop.

A long strip of fascia—the linea alba—creates the separation line down the middle of your abs and helps prevent your abs from being ripped apart by your obliques.

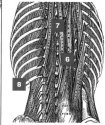

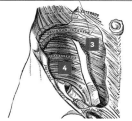

Your deepest abdominal muscle is the transverse abdominis [4]. This muscle lies beneath your rectus abdominis and obliques, and its job is to pull your abdominal wall inward—as when you're sucking in your gut.

YOUR CORE, DEFINED

While it's common to use the words core and abs interchangeably, it's not entirely accurate. That's because the term core actually describes the more than two dozen abdominal, lower-back, and hip muscles that stabilize your spine to keep your torso upright. What's more, your core muscles allow you to bend your torso forward, back, and from side to side, as well as rotate. As a result, your core is critical in everything you do—except, perhaps, sleeping.

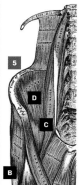

Hips

A group of muscles on the fronts of your hips, known as your hip flexors [5], also play a valuable role in core strength. The reason: They originate on either your spine or pelvis, an area that you might call the ground floor of your core. A number of muscles qualify as hip flexors, but the main ones are the tensor fascia latae [B], psoas [C], and iliacus [D]. As the name suggests, these muscles allow you to flex your hips. To visualize, imagine raising your upper legs toward your chest. You can target these muscles with exercises such as the reverse crunch and the hanging leg raise.

Lower Back

There are many lower-back muscles that contribute to your core strength, but for simplicity's sake, the main ones are your erector spinae (shown as sacrospinalis) [6], multifidus [7], and quadratus lumborum [8]. Collectively, these muscles help keep your spine stable and also allow it to bend backward and to the side. They're best trained with stability exercises such as the plank, side plank, and the prone cobra, and also with any exercise that requires you to bend or pull. What's more, even though your gluteus maximus is technically a hip muscle—and was covered in depth in Chapter 6—it's also worth mentioning here. That's because it's attached to your lower back by connective tissue and, therefore, works in conjunction with your other core muscles.

Core |

In this chapter, you'll find 68 exercises that target the muscles of your core. You'll notice that certain exercises have been designated as a Main Move. Master this basic version of an exercise, and you'll be able to do all its variations with flawless form.

STABILITY EXERCISES

These exercises improve your ability to stabilize your spine. This is essential for lower-back health and peak performance in any sport. But don't worry: Stability exercises are also highly effective at working the abdominal muscles that are most visible—including the ones that make up your six-pack.

MAIN MOVE
Plank

- Start to get into a pushup position, but bend your elbows and rest your weight on your forearms instead of on your hands.

- Your body should form a straight line from your shoulders to your ankles.

- Brace your core by contracting your abs as if you were about to be punched in the gut.

- Hold this position for 30 seconds—or as directed—while breathing deeply.

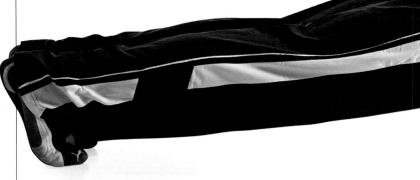

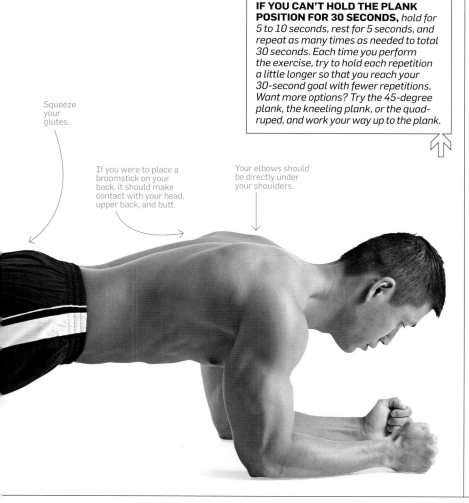

IF YOU CAN'T HOLD THE PLANK POSITION FOR 30 SECONDS, *hold for 5 to 10 seconds, rest for 5 seconds, and repeat as many times as needed to total 30 seconds. Each time you perform the exercise, try to hold each repetition a little longer so that you reach your 30-second goal with fewer repetitions. Want more options? Try the 45-degree plank, the kneeling plank, or the quadruped, and work your way up to the plank.*

Squeeze your glutes.

If you were to place a broomstick on your back, it should make contact with your head, upper back, and butt.

Your elbows should be directly under your shoulders.

MUSCLE MISTAKE
You Think Crunches Make You Thin

Researchers at the University of Virginia found that it takes 250,000 crunches to burn 1 pound of fat—that's 100 crunches a day for 7 years. So simply working the muscles buried beneath your gut won't give you a six-pack. Your best strategy for fat loss is to work all of the muscles of your body, spending most of your time training the big muscles of your lower body and back. That's because the more muscles you work, the more calories you burn.

Core | STABILITY EXERCISES

VARIATION #1
45-Degree Plank
- Place your forearms on a bench instead of on the floor.

The plank is easier when you place your elbows on a bench, since you don't have to support as much of your body weight.

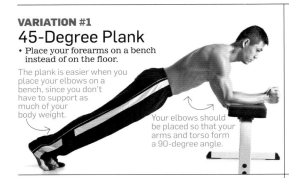

Your elbows should be placed so that your arms and torso form a 90-degree angle.

VARIATION #2
Kneeling Plank
- Instead of performing the exercise with your legs straight, bend your knees so that they help support your body weight.

Your body should form a straight line from your shoulders to your knees.

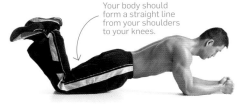

VARIATION #3
Elevated-Feet Plank
- Place both feet on a bench.

Elevating your feet increases the difficulty of the exercise.

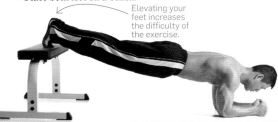

VARIATION #4
Single-Leg Elevated-Feet Plank
- Place one foot on a bench and hold your other foot a couple of inches above it. Switch legs each set.

VARIATION #5
Extended Plank
- Place your weight on your hands (as you would for a pushup) and position them 6 to 8 inches in front of your shoulders.

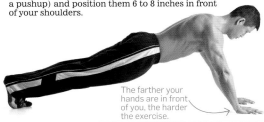

The farther your hands are in front of you, the harder the exercise.

VARIATION #6
Wide-Stance Plank with Leg Lift
- Move your feet out wider than your shoulders, and hold one foot a few inches off the floor. Switch legs each set.

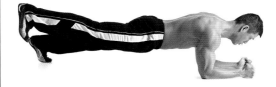

VARIATION #7
Wide-Stance Plank with Diagonal Arm Lift

- Move your feet out wider than your shoulders, instead of placing them close together.

- Raise and straighten your right arm—with your thumb pointing up—and hold it diagonally in relation to your torso.

- Hold for 5 to 10 seconds and switch arms. That's one rep.

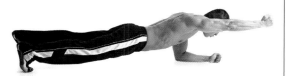

VARIATION #8
Wide-Stance Plank with Opposite Arm and Leg Lift

- Move your feet out wider than your shoulders.

- Hold your left foot and your right arm off the floor for 5 to 10 seconds, then switch arms and legs and repeat. That's one rep.

When you raise your arm and leg, focus on holding your hips and torso in place.

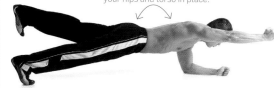

VARIATION #9
Swiss-Ball Plank

- Place your forearms on a Swiss ball and your feet on a bench.

TWICE THE ABS WORKOUT
Canadian researchers determined that your abs work nearly twice as hard when you do a plank on a Swiss ball instead of on the floor.

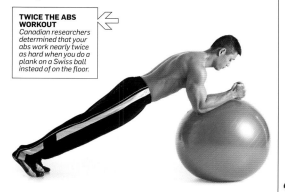

VARIATION #10
Swiss-Ball Plank with Feet on Bench

- Place your forearms on a Swiss ball.

Putting your feet on the bench raises your feet to the same level as your elbows, similar to how you would be on the floor—only the instability of the Swiss ball makes it harder to hold your position.

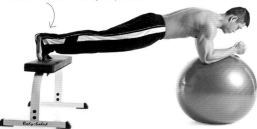

Core |

MAIN MOVE
Quadruped

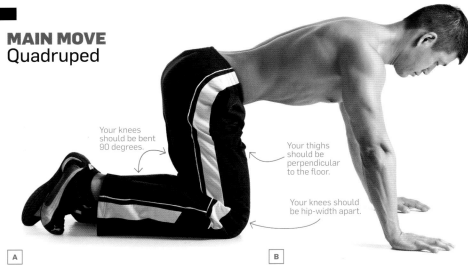

Your knees should be bent 90 degrees.

Your thighs should be perpendicular to the floor.

Your knees should be hip-width apart.

A

- Get down on your hands and knees with your palms flat on the floor and shoulder-width apart.
- Relax your core so that your lower back and abdomen are in their natural positions.

B

- Without allowing your lower back to rise or round, brace your abs as if you were about to be punched in the gut. Hold your abs tight for 5 to 10 seconds, breathing deeply throughout the exercise. That's one repetition.

VARIATION #1
Fire Hydrant In-Out

A

- Without allowing your lower-back posture to change, raise your right knee as close as you can to your chest. (Your knee may not move forward much.)

B

- Keeping your right knee bent, raise your thigh out to the side without moving your hips.

C

- Kick your raised right leg straight back until it's in line with your torso. That's one rep.

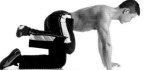

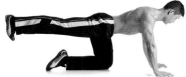

VARIATION #2
Quadruped with Leg Lift

- Without allowing your lower-back posture to change, raise and straighten your left leg until it's in line with your body. Hold for 5 to 10 seconds.

- Return to the starting position. Repeat with your right leg. Continue to alternate back and forth.

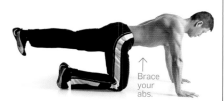

Brace your abs.

VARIATION #3
Bird Dog

- Brace your abs, and raise your right arm and left leg until they're in line with your body. Hold for 5 to 10 seconds.

- Return to the starting position. Repeat with your left arm and right leg. Continue to alternate back and forth.

Try to keep your hips and lower back still, even as you switch arms and legs.

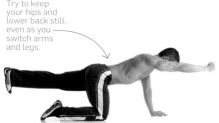

Swiss-Ball Opposite Arm and Leg Lift

- Lie belly-side down with your navel over the center of a Swiss ball.

- You should be on the balls of both feet, with your hands placed flat on the floor.

- Brace your abs, and raise your right arm and left leg until they're in line with your body and hold that position for a few seconds.

- Return to the starting position. Repeat with your left arm and right leg. Continue to alternate back and forth.

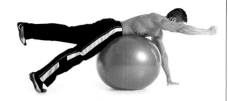

Cat Camel

- Position yourself on your hands and knees.

- Gently arch your lower back—don't push—then lower your head between your shoulders and raise your upper back toward the ceiling, rounding your spine. That's one repetition.

- Move back and forth slowly, without pushing at either end of the movement.

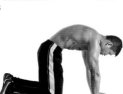

Floss Away Back Pain

The cat camel may look funny, but slowly flexing and extending your spine in small ranges of motion is a great way to prepare your core for any activity. What's more, this movement can help prevent back pain because it "flosses" the nerves of your lower back as they exit your spinal canal. This helps keep the nerves from becoming pinched, lowering your risk of painful conditions such as sciatica. It can also help free a nerve that's already impinged. A good routine: Do 5 to 10 reps.

Core | STABILITY EXERCISES

MAIN MOVE
Side Plank

- Lie on your left side with your knees straight.
- Prop your upper body up on your left elbow and forearm.

- Brace your core by contracting your abs forcefully as if you were about to be punched in the gut.
- Raise your hips until your body forms a straight line from your ankles to your shoulders.
- Breathe deeply for the duration of the exercise.
- Hold this position for 30 seconds (or as directed). That's one set.
- Turn around so that you're lying on your right side and repeat.

IF YOU CAN'T HOLD THE SIDE PLANK FOR 30 SECONDS, *hold for 5 to 10 seconds, rest for 5 seconds, and repeat as many times as needed to total 30 seconds. Each time you perform the exercise, try to hold each repetition a little longer, so that you reach your 30-second goal with fewer repetitions.*

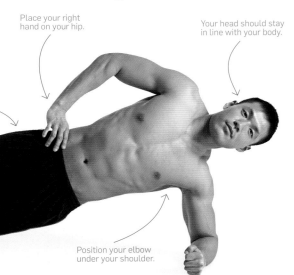

Place your right hand on your hip.

Your head should stay in line with your body.

Keep your hips raised and pushed forward.

Position your elbow under your shoulder.

VARIATION #1
Modified Side Plank
- Bend your knees 90 degrees.

Bending your knees reduces the amount of your body weight that you have to lift.

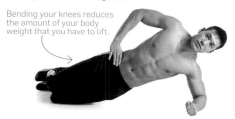

VARIATION #2
Rolling Side Plank
- Start by performing a side plank with your right side down. Hold for 1 second or 2 seconds, then roll your body over onto both elbows—into a plank—and hold for a second. Next, roll all the way up onto your left elbow so that you're performing a side plank facing the opposite direction. Hold for another second or two. That's one repetition. Make sure to move your entire body as a single unit each time you roll.

VARIATION #3
Side Plank with Feet on Bench
- Place both feet on a bench.

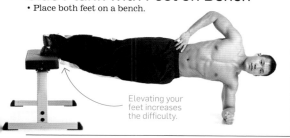

Elevating your feet increases the difficulty.

VARIATION #4
Side Plank with Feet on Swiss Ball
- Place both feet on a Swiss ball.

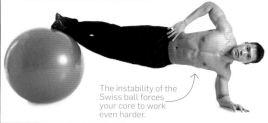

The instability of the Swiss ball forces your core to work even harder.

VARIATION #5
Single-Leg Side Plank
- Raise your top leg as high as you can and hold it that way for the duration of the exercise.

Keep your core braced.

VARIATION #6
Side Plank with Knee Tuck
- Lift your bottom leg toward your chest and hold it that way for the duration of the exercise.

Don't drop your hips or round your lower back.

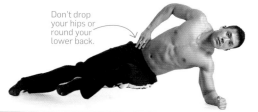

Core | STABILITY EXERCISES

VARIATION #7
Side Plank with Reach Under
- Lift your body into a side plank, and start with your right arm raised straight above you so that it's perpendicular to the floor.
- Reach under and behind your torso with your right hand, then lift your arm back up to the starting position. That's one rep.

Keeping your abs braced, rotate your torso to your right as you reach behind you with your right arm.

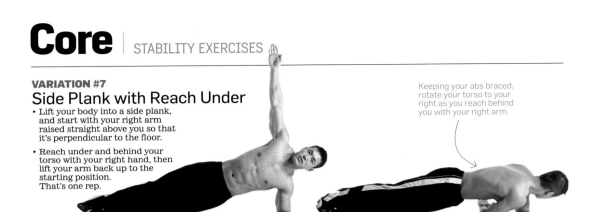

VARIATION #8
Plyometric Side Plank
- Raise your top leg slightly, and move it forward and back at an even tempo.

Moving your leg back and forth increases the challenge to your core by forcing you to stabilize your weight under conditions of varying force and movements.

Before attempting this exercise, you should be able to hold the side plank for 60 seconds.

VARIATION #9
Side Plank and Row
- Attach a handle to the low pulley of a cable machine and grab it with your right hand.
- Brace your core and raise your body into a side plank.

Your arm should be straight.

- Bend your elbow and pull the handle to your rib cage, keeping your hips pushed up and forward.
- Slowly straighten your arm back out in front of you. That's one repetition.

Resist the urge to rotate at the hips or shoulders.

The cable should be taut.

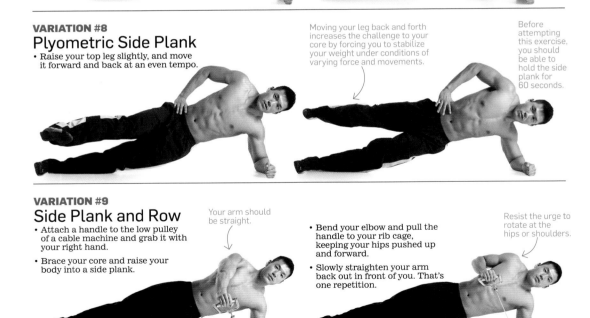

T-Stabilization

A

- Assume a pushup position.
- Your body should form a straight line from your head to your ankles.

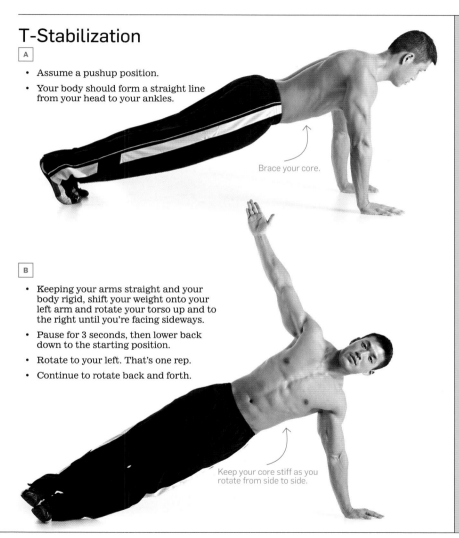

Brace your core.

B

- Keeping your arms straight and your body rigid, shift your weight onto your left arm and rotate your torso up and to the right until you're facing sideways.
- Pause for 3 seconds, then lower back down to the starting position.
- Rotate to your left. That's one rep.
- Continue to rotate back and forth.

Keep your core stiff as you rotate from side to side.

Do You Measure Up?

Researchers in Finland found that people with poor muscular endurance in their lower backs are 3.4 times more likely to develop lower-back problems than those who have fair or good endurance. And turns out, a side-plank test is one of the best ways to gauge this endurance. Simply perform a side plank for as long as you can without allowing your hips to drop or drift backward. A good score: 60 seconds. If you don't meet this standard, start focusing more on your core.

Core | STABILITY EXERCISES

MAIN MOVE
Mountain Climber

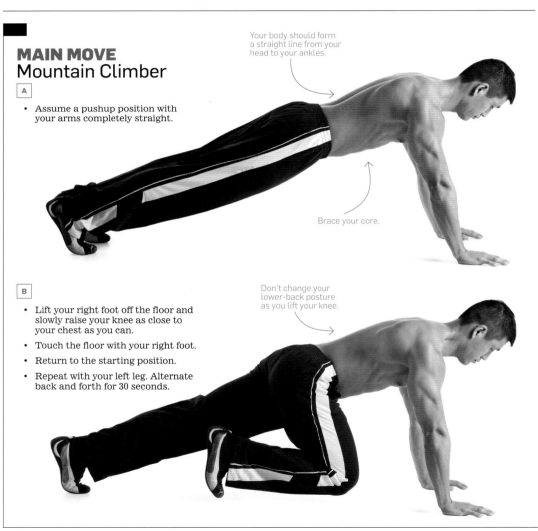

A

- Assume a pushup position with your arms completely straight.

Your body should form a straight line from your head to your ankles.

Brace your core.

B

- Lift your right foot off the floor and slowly raise your knee as close to your chest as you can.
- Touch the floor with your right foot.
- Return to the starting position.
- Repeat with your left leg. Alternate back and forth for 30 seconds.

Don't change your lower-back posture as you lift your knee.

VARIATION #1
Mountain Climber with Hands on Bench
• Place your hands on a bench, then alternate raising each knee.

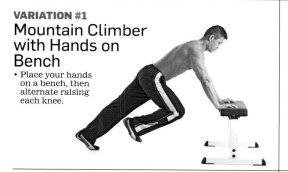

VARIATION #2
Mountain Climber with Hands on Medicine Ball
• Place your hands on a medicine ball, then alternate raising each knee.

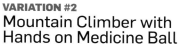

VARIATION #3
Mountain Climber with Hands on Swiss Ball
• Place your hands on a Swiss ball, then alternate raising each knee.

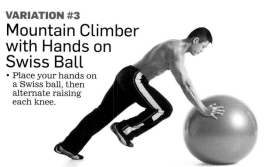

VARIATION #4
Mountain Climber with Feet on Valslides
• Place each foot on a Valslide and bring one knee toward your chest by sliding your foot forward.

As in the standard mountain climber, you can also perform this move with your hands on a bench, Swiss ball, or medicine ball.

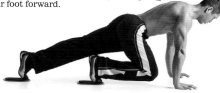

VARIATION #5
Cross-Body Mountain Climber
• Raise your right knee toward your left elbow, lower, and then raise your left knee to your right elbow.

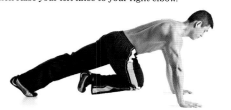

VARIATION #6
Cross-Body Mountain Climber with Feet on Swiss Ball
• With your feet on a Swiss ball, raise one knee toward your left elbow, lower, then raise the other knee.

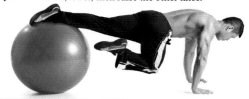

157

Core | STABILITY EXERCISES

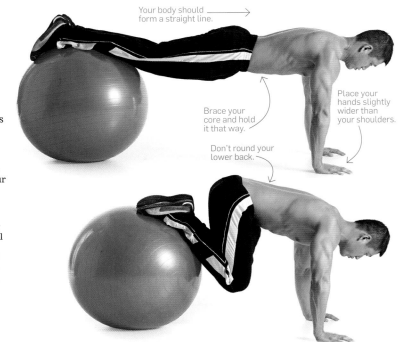

Your body should form a straight line.

MAIN MOVE
Swiss-Ball Jackknife

A

- Assume a pushup position with your arms completely straight.
- Rest your shins on a Swiss ball.
- Your body should form a straight line from your head to your ankles.

B

- Without changing your lower-back posture, roll the Swiss ball toward your chest by pulling it forward with your feet.
- Pause, then return the ball to the starting position by lowering your hips and rolling the ball backward.

Place your hands slightly wider than your shoulders.

Brace your core and hold it that way.

Don't round your lower back.

VARIATION #1
Single-Leg Swiss-Ball Jackknife

A

- Perform the exercise with just one leg, lifting one in the air as you pull the ball forward.

Don't round your lower back.

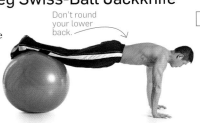

B

- Complete the prescribed number of repetitions with the same leg raised, and then do the same number with your other leg raised.

Keep your free leg elevated.

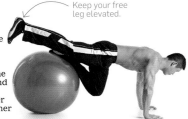

MAIN MOVE
McGill Curlup

This McGill curlup forces you to work your entire abdominal muscle complex while keeping your lower back in its naturally arched position. So it minimizes stress on your spine while increasing the endurance of the muscles. That makes it a valuable exercise for helping to prevent future lower-back pain.

- Lie faceup on the floor with your right leg straight and flat on the floor. Your left knee should be bent, and your left foot flat.

- Place your palms on the floor underneath the natural arch in your lower back. (Don't flatten your back.)

B

- Slowly raise your head and shoulders off the floor without bending your lower back, and hold this position for 7 or 8 seconds, breathing deeply the entire time. That's one repetition.

- Complete the prescribed number of reps, then do the same number with your left leg straight and your right bent.

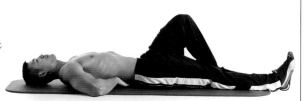

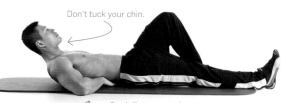

Don't tuck your chin.

Don't flatten your lower back as you curl your torso up.

VARIATION #1
Curlup with Raised Elbows

- Raise your elbows off the floor as you curl up.

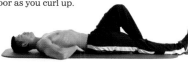

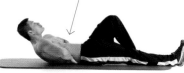

Raising your elbows makes the exercise even harder.

Core | STABILITY EXERCISES

Swiss-Ball Rollout

A

- Sit on your knees in front of a Swiss ball and place your forearms and fists on the ball.

B

- Slowly roll the ball forward, straightening your arms and extending your body as far as you can without allowing your lower back to "collapse."

- Use your abdominal muscles to pull the ball back to your knees.

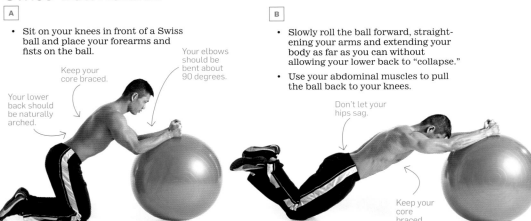

Keep your core braced.

Your elbows should be bent about 90 degrees.

Your lower back should be naturally arched.

Don't let your hips sag.

Keep your core braced.

Barbell Rollout

A

- Load a barbell with a 10-pound plate on each side and affix collars.

- Kneel on the floor and grab the bar with an overhand, shoulder-width grip.

- Your shoulders should start over the barbell.

B

- Slowly roll the bar forward, extending your body as far as you can without allowing your hips to sag.

- Use your abdominal muscles to pull the bar back to your knees.

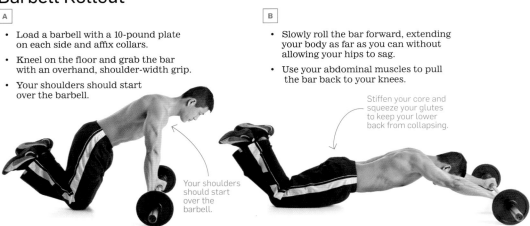

Stiffen your core and squeeze your glutes to keep your lower back from collapsing.

Your shoulders should start over the barbell.

Prone Cobra

- Lie facedown on the floor with your legs straight and your arms next to your sides, palms down.

- Contract your glutes and the muscles of your lower back, and raise your head, chest, arms, and legs off the floor.

- Simultaneously rotate your arms so that your thumbs point toward the ceiling. At this time, your hips should be the only parts of your body touching the floor. Hold this position for 60 seconds.

IF YOU CAN'T HOLD THE PRONE COBRA FOR 60 SECONDS, *hold for 5 to 10 seconds, rest for 5 seconds, and repeat as many times as needed to total 60 seconds. Each time you perform the exercise, try to hold each repetition a little longer so that you reach your 60-second goal with fewer repetitions. If the exercise is too easy, you can hold light dumbbells in your hands when you do it.*

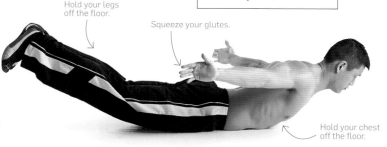

Hold your legs off the floor.

Squeeze your glutes.

Hold your chest off the floor.

Cable Core Press

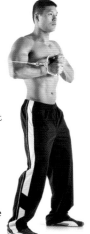

A

- With a hand-over-hand grip, grab a handle attached to the mid pulley of a cable station.

- Stand with your right side facing the weight stack and spread your feet about shoulder-width apart, your knees slightly bent.

- Step away from the stack so the cable is taut. Hold the handle against your chest and brace your abs.

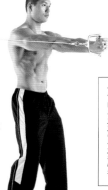

B

- Slowly press your arms in front of you until they're completely straight, pause for a second, and bring them back.

- Do all your reps, then turn around and work your other side.

THE OBJECTIVE OF THIS EXERCISE IS TO PREVENT ROTATION. *So if you're hiking up your hip or rotating your shoulders, you're using too much weight. Squeeze your abs, keep your chest up and shoulders back, and move your arms at a slow and steady pace.*

Core |

TRUNK FLEXION EXERCISES

These exercises target your rectus abdominis, a.k.a. your six-pack muscles. They also work your internal and external obliques.

MAIN MOVE
Situup

A

- Lie faceup on the floor with your knees bent and feet flat.

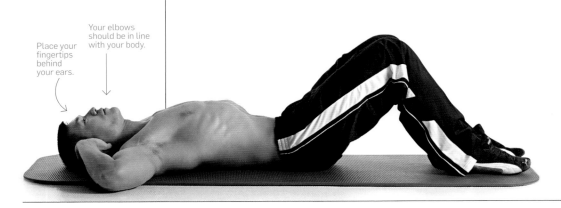

Place your fingertips behind your ears.

Your elbows should be in line with your body.

B

- Raise your torso to a sitting position.
- The movement should be fluid, not jerky—if it's the latter, you need to use a variation that's easier.
- Slowly lower your torso back to the starting position.

23

Percent reduction in heart disease risk linked to doing just 30 minutes of weight training a week, according to a Harvard University study.

MUSCLE MISTAKE
You Do Situps to Protect Your Back

While these exercises work well for building your ab muscles, they require you to round your lower back repeatedly. This can actually contribute to lower-back problems in some people, as well as aggravate pre-existing damage. So if you already have back pain, you should avoid these exercises. And as a general rule, make stability exercises the backbone of your core workout, since they've been shown to be beneficial to spinal health.

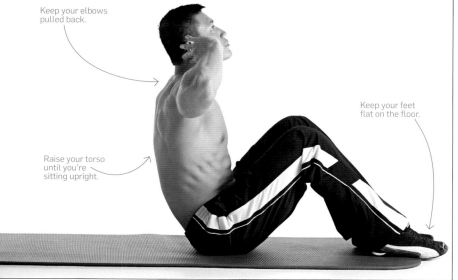

Keep your elbows pulled back.

Raise your torso until you're sitting upright.

Keep your feet flat on the floor.

Core | TRUNK FLEXION EXERCISES

VARIATION #1
Negative Situp

- Sit with your feet flat on the floor and your legs bent—as if you had just performed a situp—and slowly lower your body.

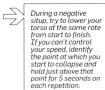

During a negative situp, try to lower your torso at the same rate from start to finish. If you can't control your speed, identify the point at which you start to collapse and hold just above that point for 5 seconds on each repetition.

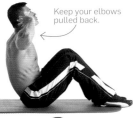

Keep your elbows pulled back.

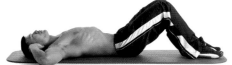

VARIATION #2
Modified Situp

- Hold your arms completely straight next to your body, raised just a bit so that they're parallel to the floor.

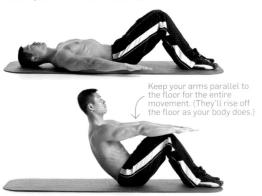

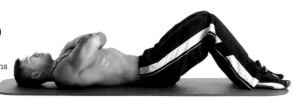

Keep your arms parallel to the floor for the entire movement. (They'll rise off the floor as your body does.)

VARIATION #3
Crossed-Arms Situp

- Perform the situp with your arms crossed in front of your chest.

- Contract your abs and curl your torso upward.

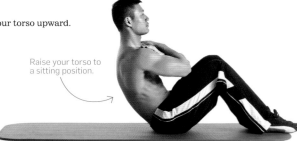

Raise your torso to a sitting position.

VARIATION #4
Weighted Situp
• Perform the situp while holding a weight plate across your chest.

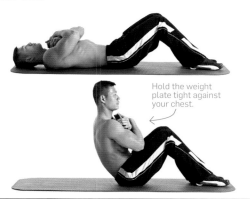

Hold the weight plate tight against your chest.

VARIATION #5
Alternating Situp
• As you raise your torso, rotate it to the left so that your left elbow touches your left knee. Lower, and on the next situp, rotate to the other side so that your right elbow touches your right knee.

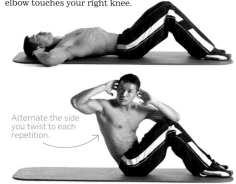

Alternate the side you twist to each repetition.

VARIATION #6
Decline Situp

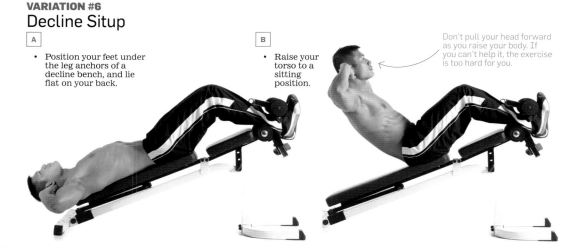

A
• Position your feet under the leg anchors of a decline bench, and lie flat on your back.

B
• Raise your torso to a sitting position.

Don't pull your head forward as you raise your body. If you can't help it, the exercise is too hard for you.

MAIN MOVE
Crunch

A

- Sit on the floor with your knees bent and your feet flat on the floor.
- Place your fingertips behind your ears, and pull your elbows back so that they're in line with your body.

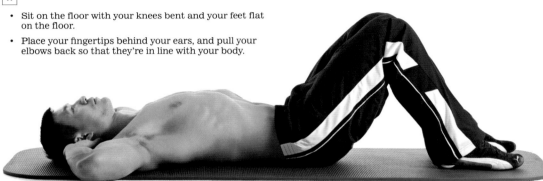

B

- Raise your head and shoulders and crunch your rib cage toward your pelvis.
- Pause, then slowly return to the starting position.

Don't pull your head forward.

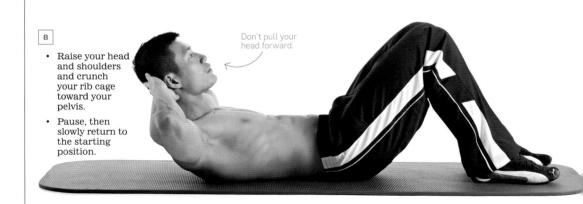

VARIATION #1
Crossed-Arms Crunch

- Perform the crunch with your arms crossed in front of your chest.

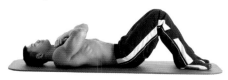

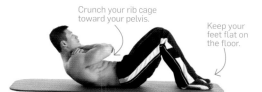

Crunch your rib cage toward your pelvis.

Keep your feet flat on the floor.

VARIATION #2
Weighted Crunch

- Perform the crunch while holding a weight plate across your chest.

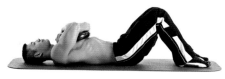

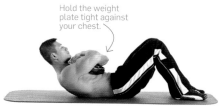

Hold the weight plate tight against your chest.

VARIATION #3
Wrist-to-Knee Crunch

- Lie faceup with your hips and knees bent 90 degrees so that your lower legs are parallel to the floor.

- Place your fingers on the sides of your forehead.

- Lift your shoulders off the floor and hold them there.

- Twist your upper body to the right as you pull your right knee in as fast as you can until it touches your left wrist. Simultaneously straighten your left leg.

- Return to the starting position and repeat to the left.

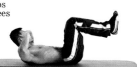

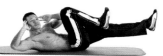

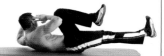

VARIATION #4
Raised-Legs Crunch

- Lie on your back with your hips bent 90 degrees and your legs straight.

- Hold your arms straight above your chest.

- Reach for your toes by crunching your head and shoulders off the floor.

- Lower your head and shoulders to the starting position.

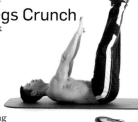

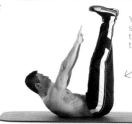

Your legs should point toward the ceiling.

Core | TRUNK FLEXION EXERCISES

MAIN MOVE
V-Up

A

- Lie faceup on the floor with your legs and arms straight.

- Hold your arms straight above the top of your head.

Your arms should be in line with your body.

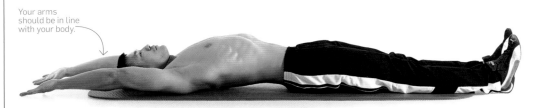

B

- In one movement, simultaneously lift your torso and legs as if you're trying to touch your toes.

- Lower your body back to the starting position.

Your torso and legs should form a V.

Keep your head in line with your body; don't crane your neck forward.

Your legs should be straight.

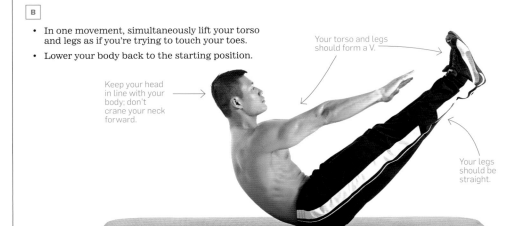

VARIATION #1
Medicine-Ball V-Up

A

- Hold a medicine ball as you do the exercise.

B

- In one movement, lift your torso and legs as you bring the ball toward your feet.

Your arms should be straight.

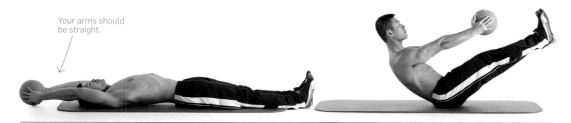

VARIATION #2
Modified V-Up

A

- Lie faceup on the floor with your legs straight and your arms at your sides.

B

- In one movement, quickly lift your torso into an upright position as you pull your knees to your chest.
- Lower your body back to the starting position.

Keep your arms parallel to the floor.

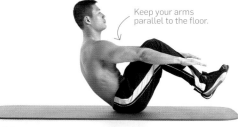

Hold your arms slightly off the floor, your palms facing down.

MAIN MOVE
Swiss-Ball Crunch

- Lie with your hips, lower back, and shoulders in contact with a Swiss ball.

- Place your fingertips behind your ears, and pull your elbows back so that they're in line with your body.

Keep your elbows pulled back.

B

- Raise your head and shoulders and crunch your rib cage toward your pelvis.

- Pause, then slowly return to the starting position.

- Don't allow your hips to drop as you crunch up.

Don't strain your neck forward.

Your feet should be flat on the floor.

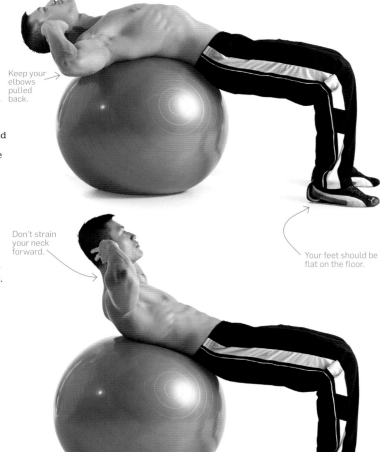

HIP FLEXION EXERCISES

These exercises target your hip flexors and your external obliques. They also work many of your other core muscles, including your rectus abdominis.

MAIN MOVE
Reverse Crunch

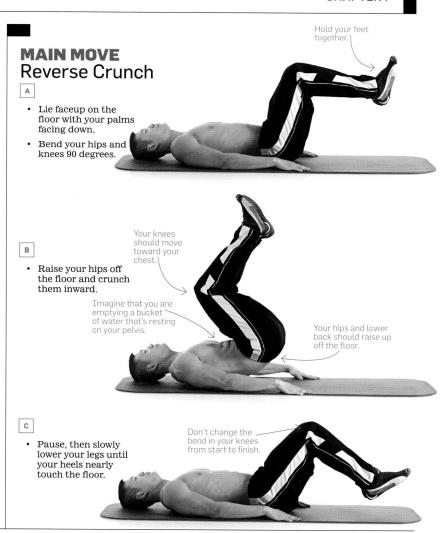

A
- Lie faceup on the floor with your palms facing down.
- Bend your hips and knees 90 degrees.

Hold your feet together.

B
- Raise your hips off the floor and crunch them inward.

Your knees should move toward your chest.

Imagine that you are emptying a bucket of water that's resting on your pelvis.

Your hips and lower back should raise up off the floor.

C
- Pause, then slowly lower your legs until your heels nearly touch the floor.

Don't change the bend in your knees from start to finish.

171

Core |

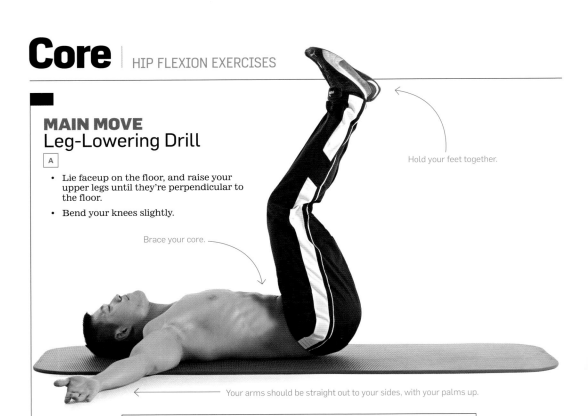

MAIN MOVE
Leg-Lowering Drill

A

- Lie faceup on the floor, and raise your upper legs until they're perpendicular to the floor.
- Bend your knees slightly.

Hold your feet together.

Brace your core.

Your arms should be straight out to your sides, with your palms up.

IF THE LEG-LOWERING DRILL IS TOO EASY:
Straighten your legs a little more. And keep doing so as it becomes easier, until you can perform the exercise with straight legs and without allowing the arch in your lower back to increase. You can also perform this on an incline bench, in a position similar to that of the incline reverse crunch.

IF IT'S TOO HARD:
Determine where the arch in your lower back starts to increase, and pause just above that point for a two-count each repetition. Then return to the starting position. You can also try the single-leg-lowering drill.

B

- Without changing the arch in your lower back or the angle of your knees, brace your core and try to take 3 to 5 seconds to lower your feet as close to the floor as you can. One trick: Press your lower back toward the floor as you perform the movement.

- Once your feet touch the floor, raise them back to the starting position and repeat.

Keep the same bend in your knees from start to finish.

When you can't stop the arch in your lower back from increasing, raise your legs back up to the start.

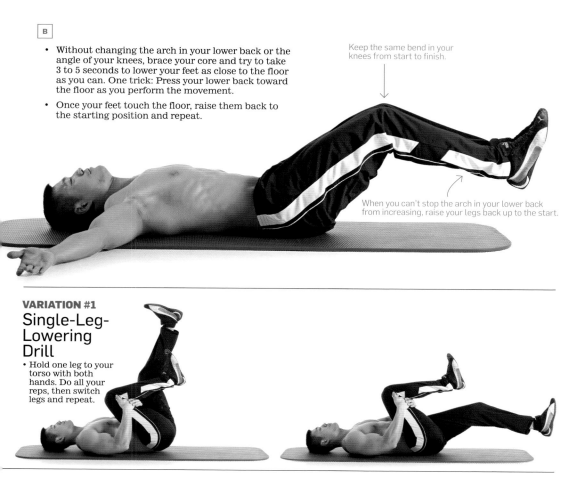

VARIATION #1
Single-Leg-Lowering Drill
- Hold one leg to your torso with both hands. Do all your reps, then switch legs and repeat.

Swiss-Ball Pike

- Assume a pushup position with your arms completely straight.
- Position your hands slightly wider than and in line with your shoulders.
- Rest your shins on a Swiss ball.
- Your body should form a straight line from your head to your ankles.

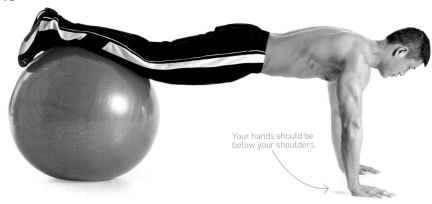

Your hands should be below your shoulders.

- Without bending your knees, roll the Swiss ball toward your body by raising your hips as high as you can.
- Pause, then return the ball to the starting position by lowering your hips and rolling the ball backward.

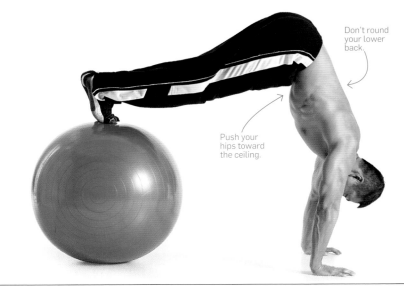

Don't round your lower back.

Push your hips toward the ceiling.

MAIN MOVE
Hanging Leg Raise

 A

- Grab a chinup bar with an overhand, shoulder-width grip, and hang from the bar with your knees slightly bent and feet together. (If you have access to elbow supports—sling-like devices that hang from the bar—you may prefer to use those.)

B

- Simultaneously bend your knees, raise your hips, and curl your lower back underneath you as you lift your thighs toward your chest.

- Pause when the fronts of your thighs reach your chest, then slowly lower your legs back to the starting position.

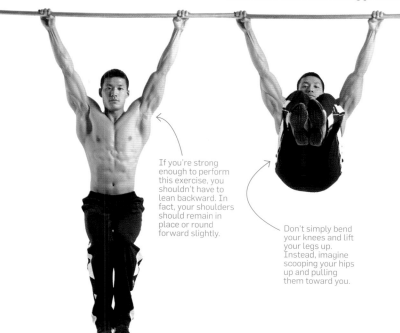

If you're strong enough to perform this exercise, you shouldn't have to lean backward. In fact, your shoulders should remain in place or round forward slightly.

Don't simply bend your knees and lift your legs up. Instead, imagine scooping your hips up and pulling them toward you.

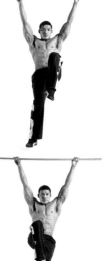

Core |

SIDE FLEXION EXERCISES These exercises target your internal and external obliques, the muscles on the sides of your torso. They also hit your quadratus lumborum, a lower-back muscle that helps you bend to the side.

Side Crunch

- Lie faceup with your knees together and bent 90 degrees.
- Without moving your upper body, lower your knees to the right so that they're touching the floor.
- Place your fingers behind your ears.

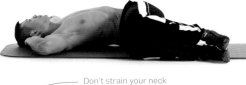

- Raise your shoulders toward your hips.
- Pause for 1 second, then take 2 seconds to lower your upper body back to the starting position.

Don't strain your neck by pulling forward with your head.

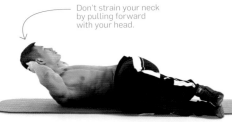

Overhead Dumbbell Side Bend

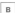

- Hold a pair of dumbbells over your head, in line with your shoulders, with your arms straight.

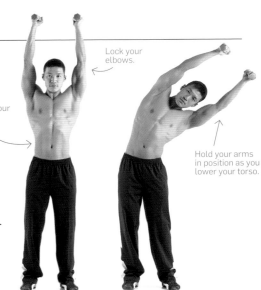

Brace your core.

Lock your elbows.

Hold your arms in position as you lower your torso.

- Without twisting your upper body, slowly bend directly to your left side as far as you can.
- Pause, return to an upright position, then bend to your right side. Alternate back and forth with each repetition.

THE BEST CORE EXERCISE YOU'VE NEVER DONE
Core Stabilization

Instead of rotating your core to move a weight, this exercise moves the weight around your core. Constantly shifting the location of the load forces your core muscles to perpetually adjust in order to keep your body stable. This not only builds your abs, but also more closely mimics the way your core muscles have to fire when you're playing sports— giving you an edge anytime you step on the court.

- Sit on the floor with your knees bent.
- Hold a weight plate straight out in front of your chest.
- Lean back so your torso is at a 45-degree angle to the floor, and brace your core.

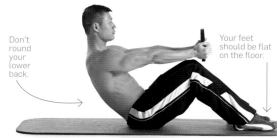

Don't round your lower back.

Your feet should be flat on the floor.

- Without moving your torso, rotate your arms to the left as far as you can. Pause for 3 seconds.

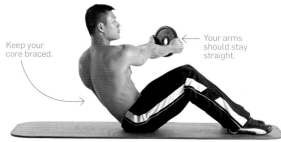

Keep your core braced.

Your arms should stay straight.

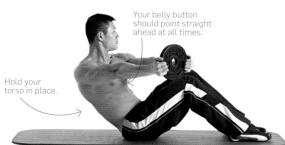

- Rotate your arms to the right as far as you can.
- Pause again, then continue to alternate back and forth for the allotted time. A good goal: 30 seconds.

Your belly button should point straight ahead at all times.

Hold your torso in place.

Total
Body

Y ou might say exercises that work your total body are ideal for anyone who doesn't like to work out. Why? Because they target several large muscle groups at once, so you can accomplish an intense heart- and lung-pumping workout—that torches calories and stokes your metabolism—with fewer exercises and in less time than ever before. Of course, for those same exact reasons, total-body moves are also great for those who *do* love to work out.

In this chapter, you'll find 9 total-body exercises. Some will look familiar, since they're combinations of exercises from previous sections. Others will seem novel. But there's one trait they all share: These movements are among the fastest ways to burn fat and build total-body muscle.

Bonus Benefits

An athletic body! Total-body exercises improve your coordination and balance. So you'll be more graceful in every activity— from tennis to running to beach volleyball.

A healthier heart! The combination exercises will convince you that the term *cardio* doesn't just apply to aerobic exercise.

Greater strength! Full-body exercises require muscles all over your body to fire simultaneously. This enhances your strength from head to toe, helping eliminate the weaknesses that may be holding you back.

COMBINATION EXERCISES

Most of these exercises are combinations of movements that appear in other chapters. Each exercise works the muscles of your upper body, lower body, and core, and is a great addition to any fat-loss workout.

Barbell Front Squat to Push Press

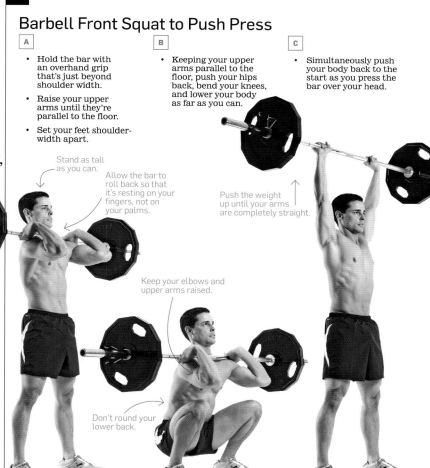

A
- Hold the bar with an overhand grip that's just beyond shoulder width.
- Raise your upper arms until they're parallel to the floor.
- Set your feet shoulder-width apart.

B
- Keeping your upper arms parallel to the floor, push your hips back, bend your knees, and lower your body as far as you can.

C
- Simultaneously push your body back to the start as you press the bar over your head.

Stand as tall as you can.

Allow the bar to roll back so that it's resting on your fingers, not on your palms.

Push the weight up until your arms are completely straight.

Keep your elbows and upper arms raised.

Don't round your lower back.

Total Body

Barbell Straight-Leg Deadlift to Row

A

- Grab a barbell with an overhand grip and hold it at arm's length in front your thighs.
- Stand with your feet shoulder-width apart and your knees slightly bent.

Bend your knees slightly and maintain that bend throughout the lift.

Set your feet shoulder-width apart.

B

- Keeping your back naturally arched, bend at your hips and lower torso until it's nearly parallel to the floor.

Don't round your lower back.

C

- Pull the bar to your upper abs.
- Pause, then reverse through each step of the movement to return to the starting position.

Squeeze your shoulder blades together.

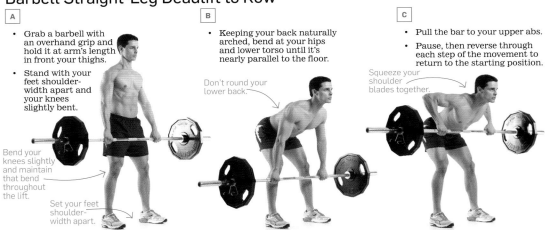

Dumbbell Straight-Leg Deadlift to Row

A

- Let a pair of dumbbells hang at arm's length in front of your hips.

Your palms should face your thighs.

B

- Bend at your hips and lower your torso into a bent-over position.

Keep your lower back naturally arched.

C

- Pull the dumbbells to the sides of your torso.

Row the weights up without moving your torso.

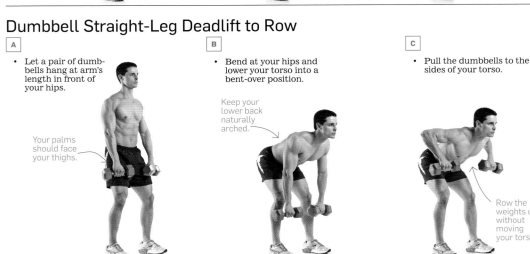

Thrusters

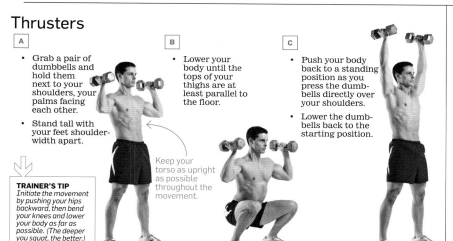

A
- Grab a pair of dumbbells and hold them next to your shoulders, your palms facing each other.
- Stand tall with your feet shoulder-width apart.

TRAINER'S TIP
Initiate the movement by pushing your hips backward, then bend your knees and lower your body as far as possible. (The deeper you squat, the better.)

B
- Lower your body until the tops of your thighs are at least parallel to the floor.

Keep your torso as upright as possible throughout the movement.

C
- Push your body back to a standing position as you press the dumbbells directly over your shoulders.
- Lower the dumbbells back to the starting position.

Dumbbell Hammer Curl to Lunge to Press

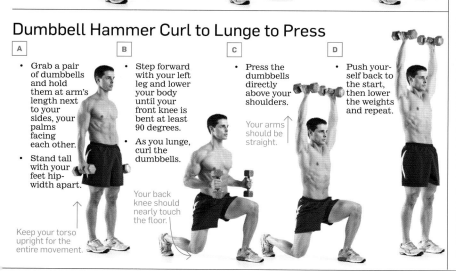

A
- Grab a pair of dumbbells and hold them at arm's length next to your sides, your palms facing each other.
- Stand tall with your feet hip-width apart.

Keep your torso upright for the entire movement.

B
- Step forward with your left leg and lower your body until your front knee is bent at least 90 degrees.
- As you lunge, curl the dumbbells.

Your back knee should nearly touch the floor.

C
- Press the dumbbells directly above your shoulders.

Your arms should be straight.

D
- Push yourself back to the start, then lower the weights and repeat.

Total Body |

Single-Arm Stepup and Press

 A

- Grab a dumbbell and hold it in your left hand, just outside your shoulder, your palm facing your shoulder.

- Place your right foot on a box or a step that's about knee height.

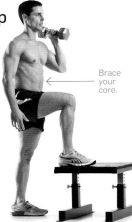

Brace your core.

B

- Push down with your right heel, and step up onto the box as you push the dumbbell straight above your left shoulder.

- To return to the starting position, lower your left foot back to the floor.

- Complete the prescribed number of repetitions with your right foot on the box and the weight in your left hand, then switch arms and legs and do the same number of reps.

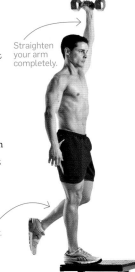

Straighten your arm completely.

Your left leg should be held in the air.

Single-Arm Reverse Lunge and Press

 A

- Grab a dumbbell with your left hand, and hold it next to your left shoulder, your palm facing in.

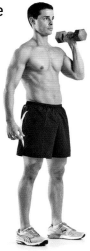

2

Times more fat people lost when they trained their entire body 3 days a week, compared to working each muscle group only once a week, according to University of Alabama scientists.

B

- Step backward with your left leg and lower your body into a reverse lunge as you simultaneously press the dumbbell straight above your shoulder.

- To return to the starting position, lower the dumbbell as you push yourself back up. That's one rep.

- Complete all your reps, then switch arms and legs and repeat.

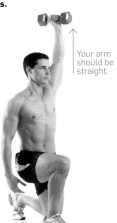

Your arm should be straight.

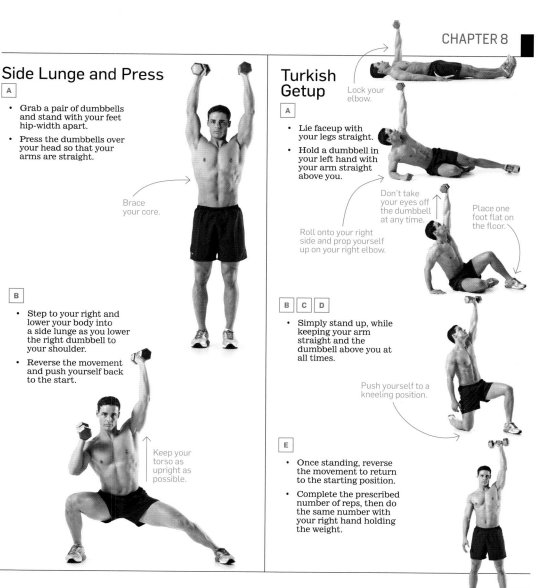

Side Lunge and Press

A

- Grab a pair of dumbbells and stand with your feet hip-width apart.
- Press the dumbbells over your head so that your arms are straight.

Brace your core.

B

- Step to your right and lower your body into a side lunge as you lower the right dumbbell to your shoulder.
- Reverse the movement and push yourself back to the start.

Keep your torso as upright as possible.

Turkish Getup

Lock your elbow.

A

- Lie faceup with your legs straight.
- Hold a dumbbell in your left hand with your arm straight above you.

Don't take your eyes off the dumbbell at any time.

Roll onto your right side and prop yourself up on your right elbow.

Place one foot flat on the floor.

B **C** **D**

- Simply stand up, while keeping your arm straight and the dumbbell above you at all times.

Push yourself to a kneeling position.

E

- Once standing, reverse the movement to return to the starting position.
- Complete the prescribed number of reps, then do the same number with your right hand holding the weight.

Warmup
Exercises

Y ou're probably tempted to flip past this chapter. After all, who has time to warm up?

The answer is everyone. You see, over the years, fitness experts have discovered that doing the right movements before a workout is like turning on the power to your muscles. Scientists believe that exercises known as dynamic stretches—what you might think of as calisthenics—appear to enhance the communication between your mind and muscles, allowing you to achieve peak performance in the gym. Translation: more muscle and faster fat loss. Surely, that isn't something you want to miss out on.

That's why this chapter provides a library of exercises that you can perform before any workout. Besides activating your muscles, the movements that have been chosen will also improve your flexibility, mobility, and posture—all critical factors for keeping your body both young and injury-free. All of this and it'll only require 5 to 10 minutes of your time.

But wait, there's more! You'll find a section on foam-roller exercises, too. These are movements that help ensure your muscles are functioning like they're supposed to. The best part: They can be done at any time—whether it's at the gym as part of your workout or after dinner on your living room floor. Just consider it the regular muscle maintenance you need to keep your body moving like a well-oiled machine.

Warmup Exercises

In this chapter, you'll find 44 exercises that help prepare your muscles for just about any activity, while also improving your flexibility and mobility.

Jumping Jacks

- Stand with your feet together and your hands at your sides.

- Simultaneously raise your arms above your head and jump up just enough to spread your feet out wide.

- Without pausing, quickly reverse the movement and repeat.

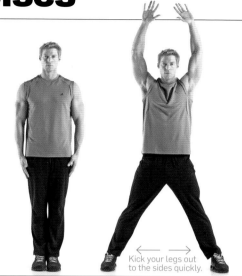

Kick your legs out to the sides quickly.

Split Jacks

- Stand in a staggered stance, your right foot in front of your left.

- Simultaneously jump back with your right foot and forward with your left as you swing your right arm forward and above your shoulder and swing your left arm back.

- Continue to quickly switch legs back and forth as you raise and lower your arms.

- Repeat as many times as you can in 30 seconds.

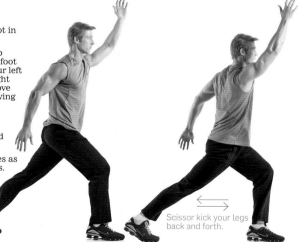

Scissor kick your legs back and forth.

Warmup Exercises

Squat Thrusts

- Stand with your feet shoulder-width apart and your arms at your sides.
- Push your hips back, bend your knees, and lower your body as deep as you can into a squat.
- Kick your legs backward, so that you're now in a pushup position.
- Then quickly bring your legs back to the squat position.
- Stand up quickly and repeat the entire movement.

As you squat down, place your hands on the floor in front of you, shifting your weight onto them.

If you want a greater challenge, do a pushup here.

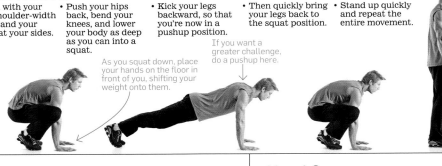

Wall Slide

- Lean your head, upper back, and butt against the wall.
- Place your hands and arms against the wall in the "high-five" position, your elbows bent 90 degrees and your upper arms at shoulder height.
- Keeping your elbows, wrists, and hands pressed into the wall, slide your elbows down toward your sides as far as you can. Squeeze your shoulder blades together.

- Slide your arms back up the wall as high as you can while keeping your hands in contact with the wall.
- Lower and repeat.

Hold for 1 second.

Don't allow your head, upper back, or butt to lose contact with the wall.

When your hands start to lose contact with the wall, slide your arms back down again.

THE BENEFIT *Enhances the function of your shoulder blades, which can help improve posture and shoulder health.*

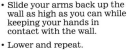

Hand Crossover

- Hold your arms so that, together, they form a straight line and a 45-degree angle with the floor.
- Your right arm should be raised, with your palm facing forward and your thumb pointing up.
- Your left arm should be held low, with your palm facing behind you and your thumb pointing down.
- Bring your arms across your body as if they were swapping positions, only keep the palm of each hand facing the same direction it was in the starting position.
- Alternate back and forth, gradually increasing the speed of the crossovers, so that you're loosely and quickly swinging your arms across your body. Do all your reps, then switch sides and repeat.

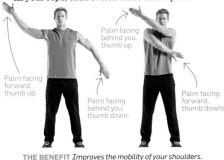

Palm facing behind you, thumb up.

Palm facing forward, thumb up.

Palm facing behind you, thumb down.

Palm facing forward, thumb down.

THE BENEFIT *Improves the mobility of your shoulders.*

Neck Rotations

- Stand tall with your feet shoulder-width apart.
- Roll your neck in a circular motion to the left 10 times (or as prescribed).
- Reverse directions, rolling in a circular motion to the right 10 times.

THE BENEFIT
Enhances the mobility of your neck.

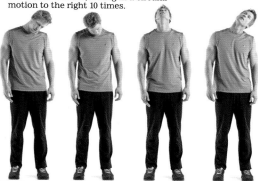

Side-Lying Thoracic Rotation

- Lie on your left side on the floor, with your hips and knees bent 90 degrees.
- Straighten both arms in front of you at shoulder height, palms pressed together.
- Keeping your left arm and both legs in position, rotate your right arm up and over your body and rotate your torso to the right, until your right hand and upper back are flat on the floor.
- Hold for 2 seconds, then bring your right arm back to the starting position.
- Complete the prescribed number of reps, then turn over and do the same number for your other side.

THE BENEFIT
Loosens the muscles of your middle and upper back.

Your arm and shoulder should touch the floor.

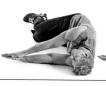

Thoracic Rotation

- Get down on all fours.
- Place your right hand behind your head.
- Brace your core.
- Rotate your upper back downward so your elbow is pointed down and to your left.
- Raise your right elbow toward the ceiling by rotating your head and upper back up and to the right as far as possible.
- Complete the prescribed number of reps, then do the same number on your left.

Bracing your abs—as if you were about to be punched in the gut—ensures that the rotation takes place at your upper back, and not your lower back.

THE BENEFIT
Enhances the mobility of your upper back, which can help improve posture.

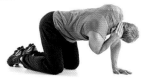

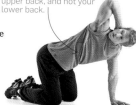

Reach, Roll, and Lift

- Kneel down and place your elbows on the floor, allowing your back to round.
- Your elbows should be bent 90 degrees.
- Your palms should be flat on the floor.
- Slide your right hand forward until your arm is straight.
- Rotate your right palm so that it's facing up.
- Raise your right arm as high as you can.
- Do all your reps, then repeat with your left arm.

THE BENEFIT
Enhances the mobility of your shoulders and upper back.

Turn your palm up.

Lift your arm.

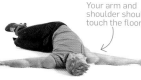

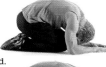

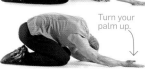

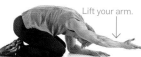

Warmup Exercises

Bent-Over Reach to Sky

- Keeping your lower back naturally arched, bend at your hips and knees and lower your torso until it's almost parallel to the floor.

- Let your arms hang straight down from your shoulders, palms facing each other.

- Brace your core.

- Rotate your torso the right as you reach as high as you can with your right arm.

- Pause, then return and reverse the movement to your left. That's one rep.

THE BENEFIT
Enhances the mobility of your upper back.

Keep your arms straight for the entire movement.

Set your feet shoulder-width apart.

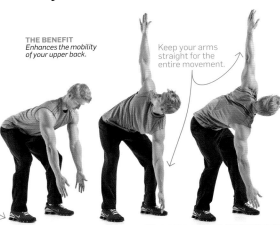

Over-Under Shoulder Stretch

- Simultaneously reach behind your head with your right hand and behind your back with your left hand, and clasp your fingers together. Hold for 10 to 15 seconds.

- Release, and repeat with your left hand behind your head and your right hand behind your back.

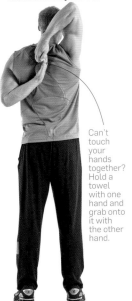

Can't touch your hands together? Hold a towel with one hand and grab onto it with the other hand.

THE BENEFIT
Loosens your rotator cuff and enhances shoulder mobility.

Shoulder Circles

- Stand tall with your feet placed shoulder-width apart.

- Without moving any other part of your body, roll your shoulders backward in a circular motion 10 times.

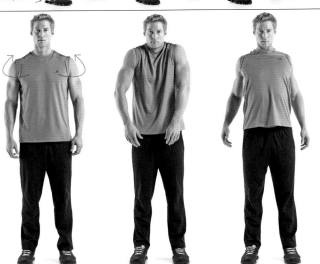

THE BENEFIT
Enhances the mobility of your shoulders.

Arm Circles

- Stand tall, holding your arms straight out to your sides, so that they're parallel to the floor.

- Start by making small circles with your arms, progressing to bigger circles. Do 10 reps forward and 10 reps backward.

THE BENEFIT
Enhances the mobility of your shoulders.

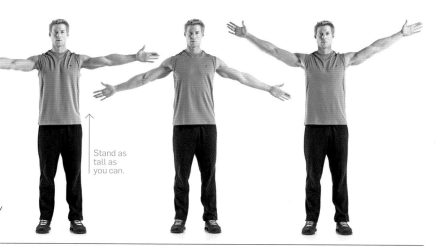

Stand as tall as you can.

Low Side-to-Side Lunge

- Stand with your feet set about twice shoulder-width apart, your feet facing straight ahead.

- Clasp your hands in front of your chest.

- Shift your weight over to your right leg as you push your hips backward and lower your body by dropping your hips and bending your knees.

- Your lower right leg should remain nearly perpendicular to the floor.

- Your left foot should remain flat on the floor.

- Without raising yourself back up to a standing position, reverse the movement to the left. Alternate back and forth.

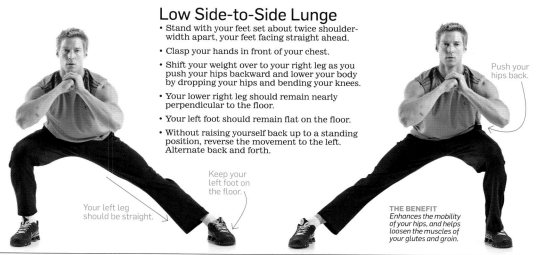

Your left leg should be straight.

Keep your left foot on the floor.

Push your hips back.

THE BENEFIT
Enhances the mobility of your hips, and helps loosen the muscles of your glutes and groin.

189

Warmup Exercises

Lunge with Side Bend

- Stand tall with your arms hanging at your sides.
- Step forward with your right leg, and lower your body until your right knee is bent at least 90 degrees.
- As you lunge, reach over your head with your left arm as you bend your torso to your right.
- Reach for the floor with your right hand.
- Return to the starting position.
- Complete the prescribed number of reps, then lunge with your left leg and bend to your left for the same number of reps.

Bend toward the same side as your lead leg.

Keep your core stiff.

THE BENEFIT
Loosens your thigh, hip, and oblique muscles.

Overhead Lunge with Rotation

- Hold a broomstick above your head with your hands about twice shoulder-width apart.
- Your arms should be completely straight.
- Step forward with your right leg and lower your body until your right knee is bent at least 90 degrees.
- As you lunge, rotate your upper body to the right.
- Reverse the movement back to the starting position.
- Complete the prescribed number of reps, then do the same number with your left leg, rotating to your left.

THE BENEFIT
Loosens your thigh, hip, and oblique muscles.

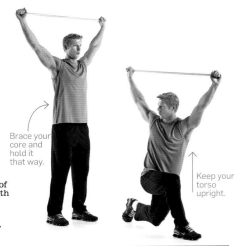

Brace your core and hold it that way.

Keep your torso upright.

Elbow-to-Foot Lunge

- Stand tall with your arms at your sides.
- Brace your core, and lunge forward with your right leg.

- As you lunge, lean forward at your hips and place your left hand on the floor so that it's even with your right foot.
- Place your right elbow next to the instep of your right foot (or as close as you can), and hold for 2 seconds.

- Next, rotate your torso up and to the right and reach as high as you can with your right hand.

THE BENEFIT
Loosens your quadriceps, hamstrings, glutes, and groin.

- Now, rotate back and place your right hand on the floor outside your right foot, then push your hips upward. That's one rep.
- Step forward with your left leg and repeat.

THE WORLD'S GREATEST STRETCH?
That's what Mark Verstegen, the famed strength coach who popularized this movement, calls the elbow-to-foot lunge.

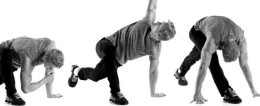

Inchworm

- Stand tall with your legs straight and bend over and touch the floor.

- Keeping your legs straight, walk your hands forward.

- Then take tiny steps to walk your feet back to your hands. That's one repetition.

If you can't reach the floor with your legs straight, bend your knees just enough so you can. As your flexibility improves, try to straighten them a little more.

THE BENEFIT
Loosens your thigh, hip, and oblique muscles.

Walk your hands out as far as you can without allowing your hips to sag.

Keep your core braced.

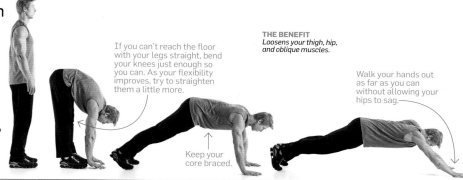

Sumo Squat to Stand

- Stand tall with your legs straight and your feet shoulder-width apart.

- Keeping your legs straight, bend over and grab your toes. (If you need to bend your knees you can, but bend them only as much as necessary.)

- Without letting go of your toes, lower your body into a squat as you raise your chest and shoulders up.

- Staying in the squat position, raise your right arm up high and wide. Then raise your left arm.

- Now stand up.

THE BENEFIT
Loosens your quadriceps, hamstrings, glutes, groin, and lower back.

Your arms should be straight.

Raise one arm straight above your shoulder, and then the other.

Keep your chest and head up.

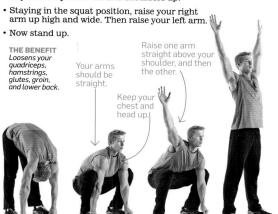

Inverted Hamstring

- Stand on your left leg, your knee bent slightly.

- Raise your right foot slightly off the floor.

- Without changing the bend in your left knee, bend at your hips and lower your torso until it's parallel to the floor.

- As you bend over, raise your arms straight out from your sides until they're in line with your torso, your palms facing down.

- Your right leg should stay in line with your body as you lower your torso.

- Return to the start. Complete the prescribed number of reps on your left leg, then do the same number on your right.

Keep your lower back naturally arched.

Your arms should form a T with your body.

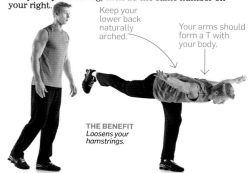

THE BENEFIT
Loosens your hamstrings.

Warmup Exercises

Lateral Slide

- Stand with your feet just beyond shoulder width.

- Push your hips back, bend your knees, and lower your body until your hips are just slightly higher than your knees.

- Shuffle to your left by taking a step to your left with your right foot and then one with your left foot. Slide about 10 feet.

- Slide back to your right.

- Repeat for 30 seconds, or as prescribed.

You should be in an athletic stance.

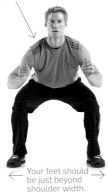

← Your feet should be just beyond shoulder width. →

THE BENEFIT
Improves the rotational and side-to-side mobility of your hips.

Walking High Knees

- Stand tall with your feet shoulder-width apart.

- Without changing your posture, raise your left knee as high as you can and step forward.

- Repeat with your right leg. Continue to alternate back and forth.

THE BENEFIT
Loosens your glutes and hamstrings.

Don't round your lower back.

Walking Leg Cradles

- Stand with your feet shoulder-width apart and your arms at your sides.

- Step forward with your left leg as you lift your right knee and grasp it with your right hand and grasp your right ankle with your left hand.

- Stand up as tall as you can while you gently pull your right leg toward your chest.

- Release your leg, take three steps forward, and repeat by raising your left knee. Continue to alternate back and forth.

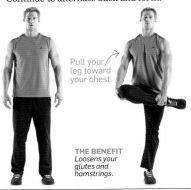

Pull your leg toward your chest.

THE BENEFIT
Loosens your glutes and hamstrings.

Walking Knee Hugs

- Stand with your feet shoulder-width apart and your arms at your sides.

- Step forward with your right leg, bend your knee, and lean forward slightly at your hips.

- Lift your left knee toward your chest, grasping it with both hands just below your kneecap. Then pull it as close to the middle of your chest as you can, while you stand up tall.

- Release your leg, take three steps forward, and repeat by raising your right knee. Continue to alternate back and forth.

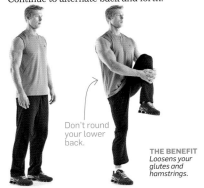

Don't round your lower back.

THE BENEFIT
Loosens your glutes and hamstrings.

Lateral Stepover

- Stand with your right side facing a bench.
- Lift your right knee in front of you, then rotate your thigh to step over the bench.
- Follow with your left leg.
- As soon as your left leg touches the floor, reverse the movement back to the other side. That's one rep.

THE BENEFIT
Enhances the mobility of your thighs and hips.

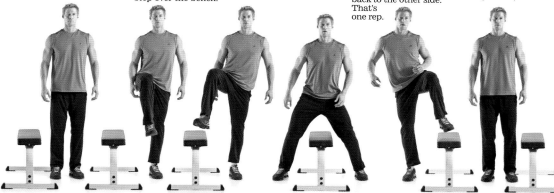

Lateral Duck Under

- Set a barbell in a squat rack or Smith machine a little higher than waist level.
- Stand with your left side next to the bar.
- Take a long stride under the bar, and shift your weight toward your left leg as you squat low to duck under the bar in one movement.
- Rise to a standing position on the other side of the bar.
- Reverse the movement to return to the starting position.

THE BENEFIT
Enhances the mobility of your thighs and hips.

You don't actually need a bench or a bar to perform the lateral stepover or duck under. Just imagine there's one there and perform the move.

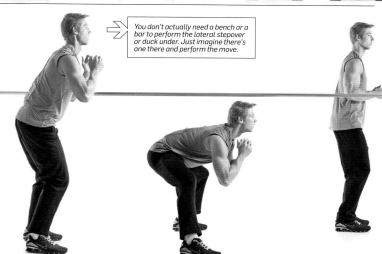

Warmup Exercises

Lying Side Leg Raise

- Lie on your left side with your legs straight, your right leg on top of your left. Brace your left upper arm on the floor, and support your head with your left hand.

- Keeping your knee straight, raise your left leg as high as possible in a straight line.

- Lower your leg back to the starting position.

THE BENEFIT
Loosens your hip adductors, or groin.

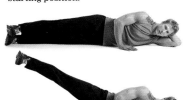

Walking Heel to Butt

- Stand tall with your arms at your sides.

- Step forward with your left leg, then lift your right ankle toward your butt, grasping it with your right hand.

- Pull your ankle as close to your butt as you can.

- Release your ankle, take three steps forward, and repeat by raising your left ankle.

THE BENEFIT
Loosens your quadriceps.

Lying Straight Leg Raise

- Lie faceup on the floor with your legs straight.

- Keeping both knees straight, raise your right leg upward as far as possible. (Imagine that you're trying to kick a ball that's hanging over your body.)

- Complete the prescribed number of reps with your right leg, then do the same number with your left leg.

THE BENEFIT
Loosens your hamstrings.

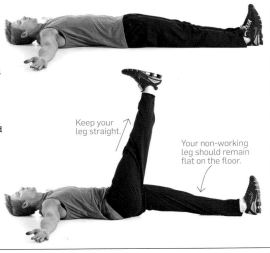

Keep your leg straight.

Your non-working leg should remain flat on the floor.

Walking High Kicks

- Stand tall with arms hanging at your sides.

- Keeping your knee straight, kick your right leg up—reaching with your left arm out to meet it—as you simultaneously take a step forward. (Just imagine that you're a Russian soldier.)

- As soon as your right foot touches the floor, repeat the movement with your left leg and right arm. Alternate back and forth.

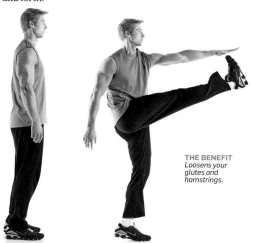

THE BENEFIT
Loosens your glutes and hamstrings.

Prone Hip Internal Rotation

- Lie facedown on the floor with your knees together and bent 90 degrees.

- Without allowing your hips to rise off the floor, lower your feet straight out to the sides as far as you comfortably can. Hold for 1 or 2 seconds, then return to the starting position.

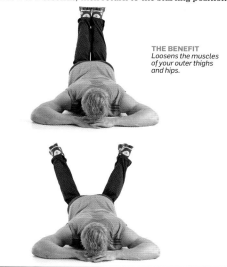

THE BENEFIT
Loosens the muscles of your outer thighs and hips.

Groiners

- Get into pushup position.

THE BENEFIT
Loosens your hip adductors, or groin, and enhances hip mobility.

- Bring your right foot forward, place it next to your right hand (or as close as you can), and lower your hips for a brief moment.

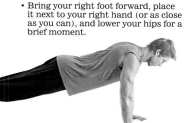

- Return to the start, and repeat with your left leg.

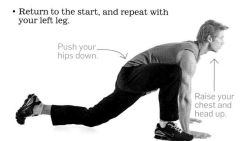

Push your hips down.

Raise your chest and head up.

195

Warmup Exercises

Ankle Circles

- Stand tall on one foot, and raise your left thigh until it's parallel to the floor. Clasp your hands under your left knee to support your leg.

- Without moving your lower leg, rotate your ankle clockwise. Each circle is one repetition.

- Complete all your reps, then do the same number in a counterclockwise direction. Repeat with your right leg.

THE BENEFIT
Enhances the mobility of your ankles.

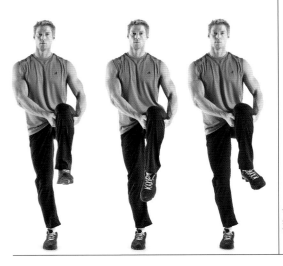

Ankle Flexion

- Place the balls of your feet on a surface that's about 2 inches high, with your heels on the floor.

- Stand tall with your legs nearly straight.

- Bend your knees and shift your weight forward until you feel a stretch in the backs of your heels. Hold for 2 or 3 seconds, then return to the starting position. That's one repetition.

THE BENEFIT
Enhances the mobility of your ankles.

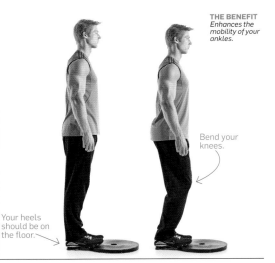

Bend your knees.

Your heels should be on the floor.

Supine Hip Internal Rotation

- Lie faceup on the floor with your knees bent 90 degrees.

- Your feet should be flat on the floor and about twice shoulder-width apart.

- Without allowing your feet to move, lower your knees inward as far as you comfortably can. Hold for 1 or 2 seconds, then return to the starting position.

THE BENEFIT
Loosens the muscles of your inner thighs and hips.

Your feet should remain stationary.

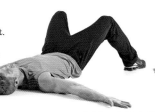

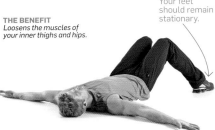

FOAM-ROLL EXERCISES

You might liken these foam-roller exercises to a deep massage. By rolling the hard foam over your thighs, calves, and back, you'll loosen tough connective tissue and decrease the stiffness of your muscles. This helps enhance your flexibility and mobility and keeps your muscles functioning properly. As a result, foam-rolling exercises are valuable both before and after a hard workout, and really, anytime you have the opportunity. Want to multitask? Pull out the foam roller while you're watching TV.

At first, you may find foam rolling to be uncomfortable. This will be especially true for the muscles that need it most. The more it hurts, the more you need to roll. The good news: Roll regularly, and you'll notice that your muscles will become a little less tender with every subsequent session. For each muscle that you work, slowly move the roller back and forth over it for 30 seconds. If you hit a point that's particularly tender, pause on it for 5 to 10 seconds.

Your main objective: Focus on foam rolling the muscles that need it the most. Trust me, you'll know which ones those are as soon as you start experimenting with the exercises that follow. You can buy your own 36-inch foam roll at most fitness-equipment stores. But in a pinch, you can substitute a basketball, tennis ball, or a section of PVC pipe.

Hamstrings Roll

- Place a foam roller under your right knee, with your leg straight.
- Cross your left leg over your right ankle.
- Put your hands flat on the floor for support.
- Keep your back naturally arched.
- Roll your body forward until the roller reaches your glutes. Then roll back and forth.
- Repeat with the roller under your left thigh.

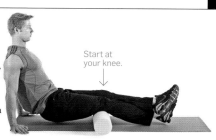

Start at your knee.

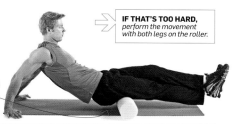

IF THAT'S TOO HARD, perform the movement with both legs on the roller.

Roll to the bottoms of your glutes.

Glutes Roll

- Sit on a foam roller, with it positioned on the back of your right thigh, just below your glutes.
- Cross your right leg over the front of your left thigh.
- Put your hands flat on the floor for support.
- Roll your body forward until the roller reaches your lower back. Then roll back and forth.
- Repeat with the roller under your left glutes.

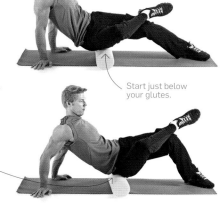

Start just below your glutes.

Roll to your lower back.

Warmup Exercises

Iliotibial-Band Roll

- Lie on your left side and place your left hip on a foam roller.
- Put your hands on the floor for support.
- Cross your right leg over your left, and place your right foot flat on the floor.
- Roll your body forward until the roller reaches your knee. Then roll back and forth.
- Lie on your right side and repeat with the roller under your right hip.

Start at your hip.

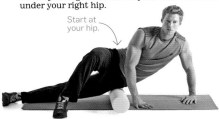

WHEN THAT BECOMES TOO EASY, *place your right leg on top of your left instead of bracing it on the floor.*

Roll to your knee.

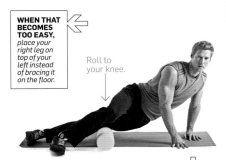

ROLL AWAY TENSION
Your iliotibial band—commonly called the IT band—is a tough strip of connective tissue that runs down the side of your thigh, starting on your hip bone and connecting just below your knee. When it comes to foam rolling, you'll probably find this tissue is one of the most sensitive areas that you can roll over, perhaps due to high tension in the band. You should make it a priority, though: Over time, an overly tense IT band can lead to knee pain.

Calf Roll

- Place a foam roller under your right ankle, with your right leg straight.
- Cross your left leg over your right ankle.
- Put your hands flat on the floor for support.
- Keep your back naturally arched.
- Roll your body forward until the roller reaches the back of your right knee. Then roll back and forth.
- Repeat with the roller under your left calf.

IF THAT'S TOO HARD, *perform the movement with both legs on the roller.*

Start at your ankle.

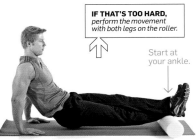

Roll to your knee.

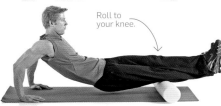

Quadriceps-and-Hip-Flexors Roll

- Lie facedown on the floor with a foam roller positioned above your right knee.
- Cross your left leg over your right ankle and place your elbows on the floor for support.
- Roll your body backward until the roller reaches the top of your right thigh.
- Then roll back and forth.
- Repeat with the roller under your left thigh.

IF THAT'S TOO HARD, *perform the movement with both thighs on the roller.*

Start at your knee.

Roll to the top of your thigh.

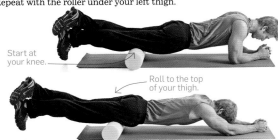

Groin Roll

- Lie facedown on the floor.

- Place a foam roller parallel to your body.

- Put your elbows on the floor for support.

- Position your right thigh nearly perpendicular to your body, with the inner portion of your thigh, just above the level of your knee, resting on top of the roller.

- Roll your body toward the right until the roller reaches your pelvis. Then roll back and forth.

- Repeat with the roller under your left thigh.

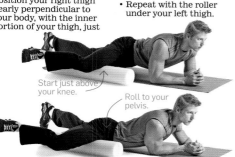

Start just above your knee.

Roll to your pelvis.

Upper-Back Roll

- Lie faceup with a foam roller under your mid back, at the bottoms of your shoulder blades.

- Clasp your hands behind your head and pull your elbows toward each other.

- Raise your hips off the floor slightly.

- Slowly lower your head and upper back downward, so that your upper back bends over the foam roller.

- Raise back to the start and roll forward a couple of inches—so that the roller sits higher under your upper back—and repeat.

- Roll forward one more time and do it again. That's one rep.

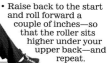

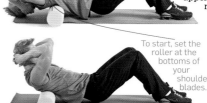

To start, set the roller at the bottoms of your shoulder blades.

Lower-Back Roll

- Lie faceup with a foam roller under your mid back.

- Cross your arms over your chest.

- Your knees should be bent, with your feet flat on the floor.

- Raise your hips off the floor slightly.

- Roll back and forth over your lower back.

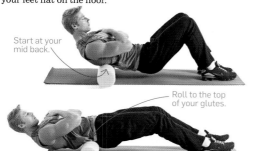

Start at your mid back.

Roll to the top of your glutes.

Shoulder-Blades Roll

- Lie faceup with a foam roller under your upper back, at the tops of your shoulder blades.

- Cross your arms over your chest.

- Your knees should be bent, with your feet flat on the floor.

- Raise your hips so they're slightly elevated off the floor.

- Roll back and forth over your shoulder blades and your mid and upper back.

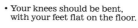

Start at the tops of your shoulder blades.

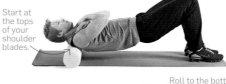

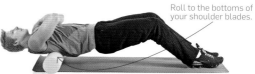

Roll to the bottoms of your shoulder blades.

Chapter 10:
The Best Workouts for Everything

YOUR COMPLETE GUIDE
TO TRANSFORMING YOUR BODY

Here are the blueprints for the body you want.

Whether your goal is to pack on pounds of muscle, skyrocket your strength, or lose your gut for good, there's a workout for you. In fact, there are lots of workouts. That's because I've enlisted the world's top fitness experts to create cutting-edge plans for just about everything—including a bigger bench and faster fat loss. There's also a workout for every lifestyle. Too busy for the gym? Try an intense 15-minute routine. Always on the road? There's a body-weight workout you can do in your room. Can't do even one pullup? The Ultimate Chinup Workout on page 210 is what you need.

Simply choose one of the plans that follow and use the instructions on page 203 to make sure you do it right. (And for even more routines, downloaded straight to your iPhone or Android, check out the *Men's Health Workouts* app from the iTunes store and in GooglePlay.)

Now get to work. Your new body is waiting.

Best Workouts for Everything

Before You Start: What You Need to Know

Use these instructions to ensure you understand how to do each workout in this chapter.

How to Do These Workouts

• Always perform the exercises in the order shown.

• When you see a number without a letter next to it—such as "1" or "4"—perform the exercise as a straight set. That is, do one set of the exercise, rest for the prescribed amount of time, and then do another set. Complete all sets of this exercise before moving on to the next.

• When you see a number with a letter next to it—such as "2A"—it indicates that the exercise is to be performed as part of a group of exercises. (A group of exercises all share the same number, but will each have a different letter, for example: 1A, 1B, and 1C.) Do one set of the exercise, rest for the prescribed amount of time, and then do one set of the next exercise in the group. For instance, if you see 2A and 2B in a workout, complete one set of Exercise 2A, rest for the prescribed amount of time, then do one set of Exercise 2B, and rest again. Repeat until you've completed all of your sets for each exercise. Follow this procedure regardless of how many exercises are in a group.

• You'll notice that sometimes the prescribed rest period is actually "0"—zero seconds. That means you're not to rest between movements; move directly to the next exercise.

• When a duration (for example, 30 seconds) is given for the number of reps, simply perform the exercise for the prescribed time. So if it's a plank or side plank, hold the position for the duration of the set. If it's an exercise in which you normally do repetitions, complete as many reps as you can in the given time period.

• The acronym AMAP stands for *"as many as possible."* So when AMAP is indicating the number of repetitions you should do, it means that you're to complete as many repetitions as you can. When it's indicating the number of sets you do, complete as many sets as you can in the given time frame.

• The acronym ALAP stands for *"as little as possible."* So when ALAP is indicating your rest period, it means that you're to rest only as long as you feel you need. Basically, catch your breath and get back to work.

Best Workouts

The Best Body-Weight Workouts

You don't need a gym membership to sculpt a great body. In fact, you don't even need equipment. Build muscle and burn fat anywhere with these super-simple body-weight workouts.

Workout 1

If any of the first four exercises are too hard, feel free to substitute the variation of the movement that allows you to perform the prescribed number of reps. Likewise, if you find an exercise is too easy, use a harder variation instead.

For the floor Y-T-I raises, do 10 repetitions of each letter. That is, do 10 reps of the floor Y raise, followed by 10 reps of the floor T raise and 10 reps of the floor I raise.

EXERCISE	SETS	REPS	REST
1. Body-weight Bulgarian split squat (page 107)	3	10–12	1 min
2A. Pushup (page 4)	3	12–15	1 min
2B. Hip raise (page 120)	3	12–15	1 min
3A. Side plank (page 152)	3	30-sec hold	30 sec
3B. Floor Y-T-I raises (pages 30 to 33)	3	10	30 sec

Workout 2

For the iso-explosive jump squat and the iso-explosive pushup, make sure to hold the down position for 5 seconds each repetition.

EXERCISE	SETS	REPS	REST
1. Iso-explosive body-weight jump squat (page 96)	4	6–8	1 min
2A. Iso-explosive pushup (page 12)	3	6–8	1 min
2B. Single-leg hip raise (page 124)	3	12–15	1 min
3A. Inverted shoulder press (page 62)	3	AMAP	1 min
3B. Prone cobra (page 161)	2	1-min hold	1 min

Workout 3

EXERCISE	SETS	REPS	REST
1A. Jumping jacks (page 185)	2–5	30 sec	0
1B. Prisoner squat (page 94)	2–5	20	0
1C. Close-hands pushup (page 8)	2–5	20	0
1D. Walking dumbbell lunge (page 109)	2–5	12	0
1E. Mountain climber (page 156)	2–5	10	0
1F. Inverted hamstring (page 191)	2–5	8	0
1G. T-pushup (page 11)	2–5	8	0
1H. Run in place	2–5	30 sec	0

The first time you try this routine, do two sets of each exercise. In future workouts, work your way up to five sets for each.

Best Workouts

The Best Three-Exercise Workouts

Build muscle fast with these "three and out" workouts from Bill Hartman, PT, CSCS. They include only what Hartman calls "big" exercises—those that work multiple muscle groups. There's one exercise for your lower body, and pushing and pulling exercises for your upper body. Do all three for the best results in the least amount of time.

How to Do These Workouts

- Choose one exercise from each category: Big Lower Body, Big Pull, and Big Push.
- Perform the three exercises as a circuit, doing one set of each in succession, resting as prescribed.
- Complete a total of four or five circuits, 3 days a week. Rest at least a day between sessions.

Exercise 1	Exercise 2	Exercise 3
BIG LOWER BODY	**BIG PULL**	**BIG PUSH**
• Do six to eight repetitions. • Rest for 75 seconds. • Move on to Exercise 2.	• Do six to eight repetitions. • Rest for 75 seconds. • Move on to Exercise 3.	• Do six to eight repetitions. • Rest for 60 seconds. • Go back to Exercise 1, and repeat until you've completed four or five circuits.
Barbell squat (page 100)	Chinup (page 46)	Barbell shoulder press (page 56)
Dumbbell squat (page 103)	Pullup (page 49)	Dumbbell shoulder press (page 59)
Barbell front squat (page 101)	Mixed-grip chinup (page 47)	Barbell push press (page 58)
Goblet squat (page 104)	Barbell row (page 34)	Barbell bench press (page 14)
Barbell deadlift (page 130)	Dumbbell row (page 36)	Dumbbell bench press (page 18)
Dumbbell deadlift (page 132)	Cable row (page 42)	Incline barbell bench press (page 16)
Barbell split squat (page 106)	Lat pulldown (page 50)	Incline dumbbell bench press (page 20)
Dumbbell split squat (page 106)	30-degree lat pulldown (page 52)	Weighted pushup (page 7)

Create Your Own Fat-Loss Workout

Now you can lose fat your way, thanks to Craig Rasmussen, CSCS, who has designed a cutting-edge flab-busting workout that allows you to choose the exercises. Think of it as DIY fat loss: Just plug and play—and watch your gut melt away.

How to Do This Workout

• Select your exercises using the guidelines provided on pages 208 and 209.

• Three days a week, alternate between Workout A and Workout B, resting for at least a day after each session. So if you plan to lift on Monday, Wednesday, and Friday, you'd do Workout A on Monday, Workout B on Wednesday, and Workout A again on Friday. The next week, you'd do Workout B on Monday and Friday, and Workout A on Wednesday.

• Do the exercises in the order shown. For each exercise, use the heaviest weight that allows you to complete all of the prescribed repetitions.

• Perform Exercise 1 as a straight set. That is, complete all of your sets of that movement before moving on to Exercise 2A. Rest for 1 minute after each set.

• Perform Exercises 2A and 2B as a pair. Do one set of Exercise 2A, rest for 1 minute, then do one set of Exercise 2B. Rest for 1 minute again, then repeat until you've completed all three sets of both exercises. Then move on to Exercise 3A.

• Perform Exercises 3A and 3B as a pair. Do one set of exercise 3A, rest for 1 minute, then do one set of Exercise 3B. Rest for 1 minute again, then repeat until you've completed all three sets of both exercises. Then move on to your Cardio Workout.

• Do the Cardio Workout immediately after each Weight Workout.

• Prior to each workout, complete a 5- to 10-minute warmup. Use the "Warmup" guide starting on page 184 to design a routine you enjoy.

About the Expert
Craig Rasmussen, CSCS, is a performance coach at Results Fitness in Santa Clarita, California. He's been helping clients lose fat and improve athletic performance for more than 8 years.

Best Workouts

Workout A

EXERCISES	SETS	REPS	REST
1. Core (Chapter 7)	3	12	1 min
2A. Glutes and hamstrings (Chapter 6)	3	12	1 min
2B. Upper back (Chapter 2)	3	12	1 min
3A. Quadriceps (Chapter 5)	3	12	1 min
3B. Chest (Chapter 1)	3	12	1 min

- **Exercise 1: Core** Choose any core exercise (Chapter 7) from the section labeled "Stability Exercises" (page 146). The plank (page 146), side plank (page 152), mountain climber (page 156), and Swiss-ball jackknife (page 158) are all great choices. *Note:* If the exercise—such as a plank or side plank—is done for "time" instead of "reps," simply hold it for the amount of time suggested in the exercise instructions. That's one set.
- **Exercise 2A: Glutes and Hamstrings** Choose any glutes/hamstrings exercise (Chapter 6) in which you work one leg at a time. This might be a single-leg barbell straight-leg deadlift (page 136), a single-leg hip raise (page 124), or a dumbbell stepup (page 141).
- **Exercise 2B: Upper Back** Choose any back exercise (Chapter 2) from the section labeled "Upper Back" (pages 28 to 45). So that's any variation of the dumbbell row (pages 36 to 39), barbell row (pages 34 to 35), or cable row (pages 42 to 45).
- **Exercise 3A: Quadriceps** Choose any quadriceps exercise (Chapter 5) in which you work both legs at the same time. This will be a version of the squat, such as the dumbbell squat (page 103), goblet squat (page 104), or barbell front squat (page 101).
- **Exercise 3B. Chest** Choose any chest exercise (Chapter 1). For example, you might choose a variation of the pushup (pages 4 to 13), a dumbbell bench press (pages 18 to 21), or a Swiss-ball dumbbell fly (page 23).

CARDIO WORKOUT

- Choose any "Finishers" from "The Fastest Cardio Workouts of All Time" (page 214) or any of the cardio workouts that accompany other routines in this chapter.

Workout B

EXERCISES	SETS	REPS	REST
1. Core (Chapter 7)	3	12	1 min
2A. Quadriceps (Chapter 5)	3	12	1 min
2B. Lats (Chapter 2)	3	12	1 min
3A. Glutes and Hamstrings (Chapter 6)	3	12	1 min
3B. Shoulders (Chapter 3)	3	12	1 min

- **Exercise 1: Core** Choose any core exercise (Chapter 7) from the section labeled "Stability Exercises" (page 146). The plank (page 146), side plank (page 152), mountain climber (page 156), and Swiss-ball jackknife (page 158) are all great choices. *Note:* If the exercise—such as a plank or side plank—is done for "time" instead of "reps," simply hold it for the amount of time suggested in the exercise instructions. That's one set.
- **Exercise 2A: Quadriceps** Choose any quadriceps exercise (Chapter 5) in which you work one leg at a time. This will be any version of the dumbbell lunge (pages 108 to 113), dumbbell split squat (page 106), or a single-leg squat (page 98).
- **Exercise 2B: Lats** Choose any back exercise (Chapter 2) from the section labeled "Lats" (pages 46 to 52). For example, you could choose any version of the chinup (pages 46 to 49), pullup (page 47), or lat pulldown (pages 50 to 52).
- **Exercise 3A: Glutes and Hamstrings** Choose any glutes/hamstrings exercise (Chapter 6) in which you work both legs at the same time. This might be a barbell deadlift (page 130), a dumbbell straight-leg deadlift (page 137), or a Swiss-ball hip raise and leg curl (page 127).
- **Exercise 3B: Shoulders** Choose any shoulder exercise (Chapter 3), such as the dumbbell shoulder press (page 59), lateral raise (page 64), or scaption and shrug (page 67).

CARDIO WORKOUT

Choose any "Finishers" from "The Fastest Cardio Workouts of All Time" (page 214) or any of the cardio workouts that accompany other routines in this chapter.

Best Workouts

The Ultimate Chinup Workout

Whether you can't yet manage a single chinup or simply want
to break out of your eight-rep rut, this training guide from
Alwyn Cosgrove, CSCS, will provide the right plan for your body.

If you can't do more than one chinup . . .

EXERCISE 1: Band-Assisted Chinup
What to do: Do two sets of six repetitions, resting for
60 seconds between sets, before moving on to Exercise 2.

EXERCISE 2: Negative Chinup
What to do: Do two sets, resting for 60 seconds between them.
Take as long as you can to lower your body—you should time
yourself with a stopwatch—until your arms are straight. A key
requirement: Try to lower yourself at the same rate from start
to finish. When you're able to take 30 seconds to lower your
body, or your combined lowering time for both sets is 45 seconds,
add a third set. Complete all your sets, and then move on to
Exercise 3.

EXERCISE 3: Explosive Kneeling Lat Pulldown
What to do:

- Choose the heaviest weight that allows you to complete four
  repetitions (but not five).

- Do 10 sets of two repetitions each, resting for 60 seconds
  between sets.

- Perform each repetition as quickly as possible.

- Each week, reduce each rest period by 15 seconds.

- In week 5, do one set of as many repetitions as you can.

- In week 6, start the process over again.

When you can do at least two chinups . . .

It's time to upgrade your routine. Your best option is a
method called diminished-rest interval training. Instead of
trying to do more repetitions, you'll focus on reducing your
rest times between sets. Eventually, you'll eliminate the rest
times altogether—and as a result, you'll be able to do more
reps continuously.

What to do: Simply take the number of chinups you can
complete with perfect form and divide that number in half.
That's the number of repetitions you'll do in each set. So if
you can do two chinups, you'll do one-rep sets. If you can do
five chinups, you'll do three-rep sets. (Round up if the

dividend isn't a whole number.) Once you've determined your
repetition range, complete three sets with 60 seconds of rest
after each. Do this workout twice a week, spacing the sessions
at least 3 days apart. Each week, reduce each rest period by
15 seconds. Once each rest period is zero, do an additional set
at each workout.

Once you can do 10 chinups . . .

You'll probably be tempted to stick with the status quo—three
sets of 10 repetitions each workout, say. However, you won't
improve very quickly that way. Instead, build pure strength by
adding additional weight and doing fewer repetitions. You'll
automatically increase the number of reps you can complete
with just your body weight.

What to do: To perform this workout, you'll need a TKO dip belt
(available at elitefts.net). This is a strap that goes around your
waist and that allows you to attach a weight plate to it. Now do
the workout below. For each set, use the heaviest weight that
allows you to complete the prescribed number of repetitions. So
as the number of reps you perform decreases, the amount of
weight you use increases. Do each workout three times a week;
rest for 60 seconds between sets.

	SET 1	SET 2	SET 3	SET 4	SET 5	SET 6
WEEK 1	8	6	4	8	6	4
WEEK 2	7	5	3	7	5	3
WEEK 3	6	4	2	6	4	2
WEEK 4	5	3	1	5	3	1

Once you reach week 5, start the process over, using the same
number of sets and reps that you did in week 1 but adjusting the
weight so that it corresponds to your current strength level. You
should expect to use more weight for each set in weeks 5 through
8 than you did in the corresponding sets of weeks 1 through 4.

Build the Perfect Back

Carve your torso into a perfect V with this 15-minute routine, courtesy of Craig Ballantyne, MS, CSCS, *Men's Health* fitness advisor and owner of TurbulenceTraining.com. It fully trains your lats but really zeroes in on the muscles of your middle and upper back. These are the common weak spots that lead to poor posture. Strengthening these muscles not only helps you stand tall but also improves the stability of your shoulders. The end result: You'll be able to lift more in nearly every upper-body exercise.

What to do: Choose one movement from each exercise group (A, B, C, and D). Then do one set of each exercise in succession, resting for 60 seconds between sets. So you'll do one set of Exercise A, rest for 60 seconds, do one set of Exercise B, rest for another 60 seconds, and so on. Once you've completed one set of all four exercises, rest for 2 minutes and repeat the entire circuit two more times. Perform this workout once or twice a week.

EXERCISE GROUP A
For any of the exercises except the negative chinup, do as many reps as you can up until the point at which you really start to struggle. On each rep, take 3 seconds to lower your body back to the starting position. For the negative chinup, do five reps in which you take 5 seconds to lower your body each time.

Negative chinup (page 48)
Band-assisted chinup (page 48)
Chinup (page 46)
Neutral-grip chinup (page 49)
Mixed-grip chinup (page 47)
Pullup (page 49)

EXERCISE GROUP B
Do as many repetitions as you can up until the point at which you really start to struggle. (This is usually about two repetitions short of failure.) On each repetition, take 2 seconds to lower your body back to the starting position.

Inverted row (page 28)
Incline Y raise (page 30)
Floor Y raise (page 31)
Incline T raise (page 32)
T raise (page 32)
Incline I raise (page 33)

EXERCISE GROUP C
Do 12 repetitions of this exercise. On each repetition, take 2 seconds to lower the weights back to the starting position.

Rear lateral raise (page 40)
Overhand-grip rear lateral raise (page 41)
Underhand-grip rear lateral raise (page 41)
Lying dumbbell raise (page 42)

EXERCISE GROUP D
Do 10 repetitions of this exercise. On each repetition, take 2 seconds to lower the weights back to the starting position.

Swiss-ball Y raise (page 31)
Incline Y raise (page 30)
Swiss-ball T raise (page 32)
Incline T raise (page 32)

Best Workouts

Build Perfect Arms

The key to a great arm workout: Keep it simple. And in fact, the best approach is to save exercises that target your arms for the end of your workout. After all, your arms are involved in every upper-body exercise. So if they tire out early, you won't be able to work the muscles of your chest, back, and shoulders as hard. Try this total-arm workout from Charles Staley, author of *Escalating Density Training*. It's designed to give your arms the work they need to grow, without requiring that you ever increase the duration of your workout. Instead, you'll simply do more work in less time—a little-known secret for building your muscles fast.

What to do: Choose one biceps exercise from the Arms chapter, and one triceps exercise. For each, select the heaviest weight that allows you to complete 10 repetitions. (Just ballpark it.) Then start your stopwatch, and do five reps of the biceps exercise, followed by five reps of the triceps exercise. Rest for as little or as long as you want, and repeat. Continue to alternate back and forth in this manner for 10 minutes. At anytime, you can drop your reps as desired. So as you fatigue, you might just do a set of three reps or two reps—go by feel. However, make sure to keep track of the total reps you perform in the 10 minutes. Then, in your next workout, try to beat that number. Repeat this routine every 4 days.

The Biceps Blaster

Your biceps muscles are composed of both fast-twitch and slow-twitch muscle fibers. So the key to maximizing arm size is to make sure you work all of these fibers. Try this three-move routine twice a week for 4 weeks. It hits your fast-twitch fibers with heavy weights and low repetitions, a combination of your fast- and slow-twitch fibers with medium weights and repetitions, and your slow-twitch fibers with light weights and high repetitions. You'll perform the first exercise with your arms in front of your body, the second with your arms in line with your body, and the third with your arms behind your body, to help hit the entire complex of fibers that make up your biceps.

What to do: Do this workout as a circuit, performing one set of each exercise after the next, with no rest in between. After you've completed one set of each exercise, rest for 2 minutes, then repeat the routine one or two more times. Choose any exercise from the menu, but make sure that you don't use the same grip (standard, hammer, offset-pinky, offset-thumb) on any of the movements. And to keep your muscles growing, choose new exercises every 4 weeks. For even more variety, you can also switch the order of exercises. So you might place the Exercise 3 movement first in your workout, the Exercise 1 movement second, and the Exercise 2 movement last, and so forth.

EXERCISE 1

Choose any one of these movements, and do six repetitions.

Incline dumbbell curl (page 78)

Incline hammer curl (page 78)

Incline offset-pinky curl (page 78)

Incline offset-thumb curl (page 78)

EXERCISE 2

Choose any one of these movements, and do 12 repetitions.

Standing dumbbell curl (page 79)

Standing hammer curl (page 79)

Standing offset-pinky curl (page 79)

Standing offset-thumb curl (page 79)

EXERCISE 3

Choose any one of these movements, and do 25 repetitions.

Decline dumbbell curl (page 78)

Decline hammer curl (page 78)

Decline offset-pinky curl (page 78)

Decline offset-thumb curl (page 78)

Best Workouts

The Fastest Cardio Workouts of All Time

Strapped for time? Try these novel cardio workouts used by top strength coach Alwyn Cosgrove, CSCS, and his team at Results Fitness in Santa Clarita, California. They're actually called metabolic circuits, and they're designed to challenge your cardiovascular system and speed fat loss just like hard sprints do. The big difference: You can do these routines in your basement. What's more, they also improve your aerobic capacity, just like jogging a few miles at a moderate pace. These workouts, however, take a fraction of the time, since you exercise far more intensely.

Medley Conditioning

Do one set of each exercise below in the order shown. Perform each exercise for 15 seconds, then rest for 15 seconds. Perform as many circuits as you can in 5 minutes. One note: For the dumbbell jump squat, lower your body until your thighs are at least *parallel* to the floor each repetition, then jump as high as you can.

- **Sprints or stairclimbing**
  Rest
- **Dumbbell jump squat** (page 105)
  Rest
- **Core stabilization** (page 177)
  Rest
- **Single-arm dumbbell or kettlebell swing**
  (page 143)
  Rest

Finishers

These are quickie cardio routines that you can do at the end of each workout. They're called finishers not just because they're a great way to finish off an exercise session but also because they'll help you finish off your fat.

THE LEG MATRIX

Do one set of each exercise without resting, and keep track of how long it takes to complete the circuit. Then rest for twice that duration, and repeat once. When you can finish the circuit in 90 seconds, skip the rest.

- **Body-weight squat** (page 92): 24 reps
- **Body-weight alternating lunge** (page 109): 12 reps with each leg
- **Body-weight split squat** (page 106): 12 reps with each leg
- **Body-weight jump squat** (for fat loss) (page 96): 24 reps

SQUAT SERIES

Do one set of each exercise without resting. That's one round. Complete a total of three rounds.

- **Body-weight jump squat** (for fat loss) (page 96): Do as many reps as you can in 20 seconds.
- **Body-weight squat** (page 92): Do as many reps as you can in 20 seconds.
- **Isometric squat:** Lower your body until your thighs are parallel to the floor. Hold that position for 30 seconds.

COUNTDOWNS

Alternate back and forth between two exercises (choose either option 1 or option 2), without resting. In your first round, do 10 repetitions of each exercise. In your second round, do 9 reps. Then do 8 reps in your third round. Work your way down as far as you can go. (If you get to zero, you're done.) Each week, raise the number of reps you start with by one—so in your second week, you'll begin your "countdown" with 11 reps.

Option 1
- **Single-arm dumbbell swing** (page 143)
- **Squat thrusts** (page 186)

Option 2
- **Body-weight jump squat** (for fat loss) (page 96)
- **Explosive pushup** (page 12)

Best Workouts

Sculpt Perfect Abs

For each routine, perform the exercises in the order shown, using the prescribed sets, reps, and rest periods. The Level 1 routine is the easiest, and a good place for beginners to start; the Level 3 routine is the most difficult. For best results, complete this workout twice a week. If you start with the Level 1 workout, do it for 3 or 4 weeks, then progress to Level 2, and so forth.

LEVEL 1

1. **Plank** (page 146)
Hold the plank for 30 seconds. Rest for 30 seconds and repeat once.

2. **Mountain climber with hands on bench** (page 157)
Each time you raise your knee toward your chest, pause for 2 seconds, and then slowly lower your leg back to the start. Alternate your legs back and forth for 30 seconds. Rest for 30 seconds and repeat once.

3. **Side plank** (page 152)
Hold the plank for 30 seconds. Rest for 30 seconds and repeat once.

LEVEL 2

1. **Elevated-feet plank** (page 148)
Hold the plank for 30 seconds. Rest for 30 seconds and repeat once.

2. **Mountain climber with hands on Swiss ball** (page 157)
Each time you raise your knee toward your chest, pause for 2 seconds, and then slowly lower your leg back to the start. Alternate your legs back and forth for 30 seconds. Rest for 30 seconds and repeat once.

3. **Side plank with feet on bench** (page 153)
Hold the plank for 30 seconds. Rest for 30 seconds and repeat once.

LEVEL 3

1. **Extended plank** (page 148)
Hold the plank for 30 seconds. Rest for 30 seconds and repeat once.

2. **Swiss-ball jackknife** (page 158)
Do two sets of 15 reps, resting for 30 seconds between sets.

3. **Single-leg side plank** (page 153)
Hold the plank for 30 seconds. Rest for 30 seconds and repeat once.

BONUS WORKOUT: SAVE YOUR BACK IN 7 MINUTES

To reduce your chances of a back attack, try this workout from Stuart McGill, PhD, professor of spine biomechanics at the University of Waterloo, and author of *Low Back Disorders*. This 7-minute (or less) workout increases the endurance of your deep back and abdominal muscles, to improve spine stability and ultimately reduce lower-back stress. Do this routine once a day, every day. Simply perform the exercises as a circuit, doing one set of each movement without rest in between.

Cat camel (page 151)
Do five to eight repetitions.

McGill curlup (page 159)
Hold the curlup position for 7 or 8 seconds, then lower momentarily. That's one repetition. Do four repetitions, then switch legs and repeat.

Side plank (page 152)
Hold the side-plank position for 7 or 8 seconds, then lower your hips for a moment. That's one repetition. Do four or five repetitions, then switch sides and repeat.

Bird dog (page 151)
Hold the bird-dog position for 7 or 8 seconds, then lower your arm and leg momentarily. That's one rep. Do four repetitions, then switch arms and legs and repeat.

Calorie-Crushing Circuits

If you like to burn fat, sweat buckets, and make your muscles burn, you're going to love these "40-20" interval workouts. They're called 40-20 workouts because you'll work for 40 seconds and then rest for 20 seconds for each exercise. Be prepared: The rest is short, so you won't have a lot of time to recover between exercises. That makes this workout circuit great for improving your cardiovascular fitness while also crushing calories and torching fat.

How to Do This Workout

• Choose any of the three routines shown on the next two pages. You can alternate between them 3 days a week for a complete training plan. Or you can choose one 40-20 workout, one 30-30 workout (see pages 222 to 223), and one 20-40 workout (see pages 220 to 221) and rotate between those.

• Perform the workouts as a circuit, doing one set of each exercise in succession. For each exercise, do as many reps as you can in 40 seconds, rest 20 seconds, and move on to the next exercise. Once you've done one set of each exercise, you've completed one circuit.

• Do a total of three circuits. For more variety, you can also mix and match Workout 1, Workout 2, and Workout 3. That is, do Workout 1 as your first circuit, Workout 2 as your second circuit, and Workout 3 as your third circuit.

• Rest for 1 minute where indicated within each routine. You can also eliminate that rest entirely, if desired.

• If any exercise is too hard, use a lighter weight or choose an easier variation of the move. If an exercise seems too easy, use a heavier weight or choose a harder variation of the move.

• Prior to each workout, complete a 5-minute warmup. Choose exercises from Chapter 9 to design your warmup routine.

Best Workouts

Workout 1

After 20 seconds, switch legs.

1. Dumbbell stepup (page 141)
2. T-pushup (page 11)
3. Goblet squat (page 104)
4. Alternating dumbbell row (page 36)
5. Jumping jacks (page 185)

Rest 1 minute

6. Dumbbell straight-leg deadlift (page 137)
7. Pushup (pages 4 to 5)
8. Alternating lunge (page 109)
9. Underhand-grip rear lateral raise (page 41)
10. Mountain climber (page 156)

Rest 1 minute

Workout 2

1. Alternating dumbbell lunge (page 109)
2. Floor inverted shoulder press (page 62)
3. Swiss-ball hip raise and leg curl (page 127)
4. Incline T raise (page 32)
5. Swiss-ball pike (page 174)

Rest 1 minute

After 20 seconds, switch legs.

6. Dumbbell side lunge (page 113)
7. Alternating dumbbell shoulder press (page 60)
8. Wide-stance goblet squat (page 104)
9. Neutral-grip dumbbell row (page 36)
10. Squat thrust (page 186)

Rest 1 minute

Workout 3

1. Dumbbell split squat (page 106)

2. Pushup and row (page 13)

3. Dumbbell split squat (page 106)

4. Hammer curl to press (page 81)

5. T-Stabilization (page 155)

Rest 1 minute

6. Single-leg dumbbell straight-leg deadlift (page 138)

7. Pushup and row (page 13)

8. Single-leg dumbbell straight-leg deadlift (page 138)

9. Twisting standing dumbbell curl (page 77)

10. Squat thrust (page 186)

Rest 1 minute

Do all your reps with your left leg.

Do all your reps with your right leg.

Do all your reps with your left leg.

Do all your reps with your right leg.

Best Workouts

Body Fat Blasters

Longer isn't always better. With these "20-40" interval workouts, you'll build power and blast serious fat—while working for just 20 seconds at a time. Sure, 20-second intervals might sound easy, but they won't be if you do them right. The secret: Perform each exercise explosively. That is, do every movement as fast as possible while maintaining control and keeping perfect form. Consider that you can jog for 20 seconds and hardly be winded. But what happens when you sprint as hard as you can for 20 seconds? You're gassed. That's what you're going for with each interval in this workout. After each 20-second set, you'll rest for 40 seconds. This helps you recover more fully after each set so that you can go your absolute hardest on the next one. It's all about effort, baby. That's how you get the results you want.

How to Do This Workout

• Choose any of these three routines. You can alternate between them 3 days a week for a complete training plan. Or you can choose one 20-40 workout, one 40-20 workout (see pages 217 to 219), and one 30-30 workout (see pages 222 to 223) and rotate between those.

• Perform the workouts as a circuit, doing one set of each exercise in succession. Do as many reps as you can in 20 seconds per exercise, rest 40 seconds, and then move on to the next. For each exercise, lower your body or the weight slowly (unless directed otherwise), and then push or pull it back up quickly. Once you've done one set of each exercise, you've completed one circuit.

• Do a total of six circuits. For more variety, you can also mix and match Workout 1, Workout 2, and Workout 3. That is, you can do Workout 1 as your first circuit and Workout 2 as your second circuit, and then repeat them both two times. Or you could do Workout 1, Workout 2, and Workout 3 in succession, and repeat them one time.

• Rest for 1 minute where indicated within each routine. You can also eliminate that rest entirely, if desired.

• If any exercise is too hard, use a lighter weight or choose an easier variation of the move. If an exercise seems too easy, use a heavier weight or choose a harder variation of the move. If you get done with this workout and think "That was really easy!" then chances are you aren't putting enough effort into the routine. Increase the weights—you'll use more than you would when doing 30- or 40-second sets—or choose a more challenging variation of the exercise. And don't loaf!

• Prior to each workout, complete a 5-minute warmup. Choose exercises from Chapter 9 to design your warmup routine.

Workout 1

1. Single-arm dumbbell or kettlebell swing (page 143)

   After 10 seconds, switch arms.

2. Explosive pushup (page 12)

3. Body-weight squat (page 92)

4. Chinup (pages 46 to 47)

5. Body-weight split squat (page 106)

Workout 2

1. Dumbbell reverse lunge (page 109)

   Do all your reps with your left leg.

2. Pushup and row (page 13)

3. Dumbbell reverse lunge (page 109)

   Do all your reps with your right leg.

4. Dumbbell push press (page 60)

5. Squat thrust (page 186)

Workout 3

1. Single-arm deadlift (page 133)

   Do all your reps with your left arm.

2. Single-arm deadlift (page 133)

   Do all your reps with your right arm.

3. Close-hands pushup (page 8)

4. Alternating neutral-grip dumbbell row (page 36)

5. Body-weight jump squat (page 96)

Best Workouts

Build and Burn Intervals

To be strong and lean: For most people, this is the Holy Grail of fitness. And a strong, lean body is exactly what these "30-30" interval workouts will help you achieve. For each exercise, you'll work for 30 seconds and then rest for 30 seconds. This allows you to use heavier weights than a 40-20 workout while still keeping your muscles under tension for a significant amount of time. That's how it helps you get stronger. Because you're also limiting your rest to 30 seconds, you'll be able to do more work in 25 to 30 minutes than most people do in an hour. You'll burn more calories in less time and boost your metabolism for hours after your workout.

How to Do This Workout

• Choose any of these three routines. You can alternate between them 3 days a week for a complete training plan. Or you can choose one 30-30 workout, one 40-20 workout (see pages 217 to 219), and one 20-40 workout (see pages 220 to 221) and rotate between those.

• Perform the workouts as a circuit, doing one set of each exercise in succession. Do as many reps as you can in 30 seconds per exercise, rest 30 seconds, and then move on to the next. For each exercise, lower your body or the weight slowly (unless directed otherwise), and then push or pull it back up quickly. Once you've done one set of each exercise, you've completed one circuit.

• Do a total of four to six circuits. For more variety, you can also mix and match Workout 1, Workout 2,

and Workout 3. That is, you can do Workout 1 as your first circuit and Workout 2 as your second circuit, and then repeat them both one or two times. Or you could do Workout 1, Workout 2, and Workout 3 in succession, and repeat them one time.

• Rest for 1 minute where indicated within each routine. You can also eliminate that rest entirely, if desired.

• If any exercise is too hard, use a lighter weight or choose an easier variation of the move. If an exercise seems too easy, use a heavier weight or choose a harder variation of the move.

• Prior to each workout, complete a 5-minute warmup. Choose exercises from Chapter 9 to design your warmup routine.

Workout 1

1. Dumbbell bulgarian split squat (page 107)

   Do all your reps with your left leg.

2. Triple-stop pushup (page 8)

3. Dumbbell bulgarian split squat (page 107)

   Do all your reps with your right leg.

4. Neutral-grip dumbbell row (page 34)

5. Swiss-ball hip raise and leg curl (page 127)

Workout 2

1. Single-leg bench getup (page 98)

   Do all your reps with your left leg.

2. Single-leg bench getup (page 98)

   Do all your reps with your right leg.

3. Inverted row (pages 28 to 29)

4. Medicine-ball pushup (page 11)

5. Dumbbell straight-leg deadlift (page 137)

Workout 3

1. Dumbbell front squat (page 104)

   Do all your reps with your left arm.

2. Standing supported, single-arm neutral-grip row (page 37)

3. Standing supported, single-arm neutral-grip row (page 37)

   Do all your reps with your right arm.

4. Alternating dumbbell side lunge (page 113)

5. Decline pushup (page 6)

Best Workouts

20-Second Sizzlers

There's no way to candy-coat it: This workout is absolutely brutal. But it is brutal in a good way, of course. That's because it destroys fat, blasts every muscle, and leaves you soaked in sweat. It will push you to your limits, but also energize you for the rest of the day. What's the secret? It's based on the Tabata protocol, a famous and highly effective 4-minute training method performed solely on a stationary bike. The problem is that most people can't do the *actual* Tabata protocol without losing their lunch. But this version is modified: Instead of doing a single mode of exercise, you'll alternate between two exercises that work your muscles in different ways. Therefore, you can work out even longer than 4 minutes—while keeping your lunch where it's supposed to stay. In fact, you can do one 4-minute routine, rest for a minute, and then do a second, third, and more. Challenge yourself to go for up to 30 minutes for an awesome workout that will make your fat cells cry.

How to Do This Workout

• You can do this routine 3 days a week, or rotate it in with any of the other workouts, mix and match style: 40-20 workout (see pages 217 to 219), 30-30 workout (see pages 222 to 223), 20-40 workout (see pages 218 to 219) or Triple Set Torchers (see pages 226 to 227).

• Do each pair of exercises—1A and 1B, for instance—as a superset, alternating back and forth between the movements. Perform Exercise 1A for 20 seconds, rest for 10 seconds, and then do Exercise 1B for 20 seconds, and rest for another 10 seconds. That's one superset. Complete a total of four supersets which will take 4 minutes. Then move on to Exercise 2A and Exercise 2B and repeat. Continue in this manner until you've done all five supersets. That's a 24-minute workout. Want more? You can start from the beginning

again. Every additional superset adds 4 minutes, plus rest.

• If any exercise is too hard, use a lighter weight or choose an easier variation of the move. If an exercise seems too easy, use a heavier weight or choose a harder variation of the move.

• If you like this workout but just find it too challenging, adjust your work and rest periods. You can start by exercising for 10 seconds and resting for 20, and then progress so that you exercise for 15 sec-onds and rest for 15 seconds. This way, you can exercise your way up to working for 20 seconds and resting for 10.

• Prior to each workout, complete a 5-minute warmup. Choose exercises from Chapter 9 to design your warmup routine.

Superset 1

1A. Thrusters (page 181)

1B. Single-arm dumbbell or kettlebell swing (page 143)

← Switch arms each set.

Rest 1 minute

Superset 2

2A. Pushup (pages 4 to 5)

2B. Reverse dumbbell lunge (page 109)

Rest 1 minute

Superset 3

3A. Alternating dumbbell shoulder press (page 60)

3B. Alternating neutral-grip row (page 35)

Rest 1 minute

Superset 4

Switch arm positions each set.

4A. Staggered pushup (page 9)

←

4B. Dumbbell side lunge (page 113)

←

Rest 1 minute

Switch legs each set, or alternate legs each repetition.

Superset 5

5A. Squat thrust (page 186)

←

5B. Single-arm dumbbell or kettlebell swing (page 143)

Switch arms each set.

Rest 1 minute

Best Workouts

Triple-Set Torchers

What happens when you make fat-burning workouts fun? You guessed it: You start to like fat-burning workouts! And after having tested hundreds of workouts at the *Men's Health* and *Women's Health* gym, this style of routine—inspired by training expert BJ Gaddour—is at the top of everyone's favorite workout list. It's seriously intense, but is so quick-moving and has so much variety that it flies by even though you're getting your butt kicked. You'll sweat, your muscles will burn, and you may even curse. But you will love every minute of it!

How to Do This Workout

• You can do this routine 3 days a week, or rotate it in with any of these other workouts, mix and match style: 40-20 workout (see pages 217 to 219), 30-30 workout (see pages 222 to 223), 20-40 workout (see pages 220 to 221), or 20-Second Sizzlers (see pages 224 to 225).

• Do each trio of exercises—1A, 1B, and 1C, for instance—as a "triple set", doing one exercise after another. Perform Exercise 1A for 20 seconds, then immediately do Exercise 1B for 20 seconds, followed by Exercise 1C for 20 seconds. Then rest for 1 minute, and move on to Exercises 2A, 2B, and 2C.

Repeat this procedure until you've completed all exercises and rests for a total of 10 triple sets. That's a 19-minute workout. If you want more, just start over at Triple Set 1 and repeat as many triple sets as desired.

• If any exercise is too hard, use a lighter weight or choose an easier variation of the move. If an exercise seems too easy, use a heavier weight or choose a harder variation of the move.

• Prior to each workout, complete a 5-minute warmup. Choose exercises from Chapter 9 to design your warmup routine.

Triple Set 1

1A. Spiderman pushup (page 9)

1B. Judo pushup (page 11)

1C. T-pushup (page 11)

Rest 1 minute

Triple Set 2

2A. Dumbbell split squat (page 106)

Do all your reps with your left leg.

2B. Dumbbell split squat (page 106)

2C. Body-weight jump squat (page 96)

Do all your reps with your right leg.

Rest 1 minute

Triple Set 3

3A. Mountain climber (page 156)

3B. Squat thrust (page 186)

3C. Lateral slide (page 192)

Rest 1 minute

Triple Set 4

Do all your reps with your left arm.

4A. Single-arm neutral-grip dumbbell row (page 35)

4B. Single-arm neutral-grip dumbbell row (page 35)

Do all your reps with your right arm.

4C. Pushup and row (page 13)

Rest 1 minute

Triple Set 5

5A. Hip raise with feet on a swiss ball (page 123)

5B. Marching hip raise with feet on a Swiss ball (page 123)

5C. Swiss ball hip raise and leg curl (page 127)

Rest 1 minute

Triple Set 6

Do all your reps while pressing with your right arm.

6A. Single-arm reverse lunge and press (page 35)

6B. Single-arm reverse lunge and press (page 35)

Do all your reps while pressing with your left arm.

6C. Jumping jacks (page 185)

Rest 1 minute

Triple Set 7

7A. Staggered-hands pushup (Left) (page 9)

7B. Staggered-hands pushup (Right) (page 9)

7C. Swiss-ball jackknife (page 158)

Rest 1 minute

Triple Set 8

Do all your reps with your left leg.

8A. Dumbbell side lunge (page 113)

8B. Dumbbell side lunge (page 113)

Do all your reps with your right leg.

8C. Low side-to-side lunge (page 189)

Rest 1 minute

Triple Set 9

9A. Prisoner squat (page 94)

9B. Alternating dumbbell lunge (page 109)

9C. Body-weight split squat (page 106)

Rest 1 minute

Triple Set 10

10A. Explosive pushup (page 12)

10B. Jumping jacks (page 185)

10C. Body-weight jump squat (page 92)

Rest 1 minute

Best Workouts

The Best 15-Minute Workouts

Ready to start sculpting a leaner, stronger body? It won't take you long. Just three 15-minute weight workouts a week can double a beginner's strength, report scientists at the University of Kansas. What's more, unlike the average person, who quits a new weight-training program within a month, 96 percent of the participants in the study easily fit the quickie workouts into their lives. You can do the same, with the 4 workouts that follow—all of which are designed to build muscle while melting fat.

Workout 1

EXERCISE	SETS	REPS	REST
1A. Barbell squat (page 100)	3	15	0
1B. Pushup (page 4)	3	AMAP	0
1C. Hip raise (page 120)	3	12–15	0
1D. Dumbbell row (page 36)	3	10–12	0
1E. Plank (page 146)	3	30-sec hold	0

Workout 2

EXERCISE	SETS	REPS	REST
1A. Swiss-ball hip raise and leg curl (page 127)	3	AMAP	0
1B. Pushup plus (pages 24 to 25)	3	AMAP	0
1C. Swiss-ball jackknife (page 158)	3	AMAP	30 sec
2A. Chinup (page 46)	2–3	AMAP	30 sec
2B. Dumbbell shoulder press (page 59)	2–3	8–10	30 sec

Before You Start

If any of the body-weight exercises in these workouts are too hard or too easy, feel free to substitute the variation of the movement that allows you to perform the prescribed number of reps. Remember, each set should challenge your muscles to the point where you start to struggle but don't quite reach complete failure.

And make no mistake: These workouts aren't easy. They're fast paced and intense. So if they're too hard when you first start, go ahead and take a longer rest between sets, and finish as much of the workout as you can in the 15 minutes. In each subsequent workout, try to do a little more, until you're able to complete the entire routine.

How to Do These Workouts

• Option 1: Choose a workout and do it three times a week, resting for at least a day after each session. After 2 or 3 weeks, switch to a new workout.

• Option 2: Choose two workouts and alternate between them 3 days a week. Always rest for at least a day after each session. So you might do Workout 1 on Monday and Friday, and Workout 2 on Wednesday. The following week, you'd do Workout 2 on Monday and Friday, and Workout 1 on Wednesday. After 4 weeks, it's time to choose two new workouts.

Workout 3

EXERCISE	SETS	REPS	REST
1. Single-arm reverse lunge and press (page 182)	3	10–12	1 min
2A. Chinup (page 46)	3	AMAP	0
2B. Side plank (page 152)	3	30-sec hold	0
2C. Pushup (page 4)	3	AMAP	45 sec

Workout 4

EXERCISE	SETS	REPS	REST
1A. Single-arm dumbbell swing (page 143)	3	12	30 sec
1B. Pushup and row (page 13)	3	12	30 sec
2A. Thrusters (page 181)	2	12	30 sec
2B. Swiss-ball jackknife (page 158)	2	12–15	30 sec

Best Workouts

The Spartacus Workout

Ever wonder how Hollywood actors get in such incredible shape? It's not rocket science. But it is exercise science. So when executives at Starz asked me to create a training plan for the cast of the network's new show, *Spartacus*—in preparation for the program's January 2010 premiere—I knew exactly who to consult: Rachel Cosgrove, one of the world's top fitness experts who's known industry-wide for her ability to meld the latest in muscle and fat-loss science to achieve stunning results.

For the actors in Spartacus, we mixed old-school training equipment—such as sandbags and kettlebells—with modern variations of classic exercises, like T-pushups and the dumbbell lunge and rotation, all of which were designed to mimic the movements a Spartan warrior would need in training and in battle. (To see a video of the cast working out, go to MensHealth.com/Spartacus.) For you, we've tweaked the exercises to make the workout more gym-friendly, while keeping it every bit as effective. The final product: A cutting-edge circuit routine that will strip away fat, define your chest, arms, and abs, and send your fitness levels soaring. So you'll sculpt the lean, muscular, and athletic-looking body of a Spartan warrior—while getting in the best shape of your life.

About the Expert
Rachel Cosgrove, CSCS, is the co-owner of Results Fitness in Santa Clarita, California, and a top fitness advisor to both *Men's Health* and *Women's Health*.

How to Do This Workout

- Do this workout 3 days a week. You can do it as your primary weight workout, or as a "cardio" workout on the days between your regular weight workouts. This approach will help you speed fat loss even more.
- Perform the workout as a circuit, doing one set of each exercise—or "station"—in succession. Each station in the circuit lasts for 60 seconds. Do as many repetitions as you can in that time, then move on to the next station in the circuit. Give yourself 15 seconds to transition between stations, and rest for 2 minutes after you've done one circuit of all 10 exercises. Then repeat two times. If you can't go for the entire minute on the body-weight exercises, go as long as you can, rest for a few seconds, then go again until your time at that station is up.
- Prior to each workout, complete a 5 to 10 minute warmup. Choose exercises from Chapter 9 to design your warmup routine.

STATION 1

Goblet squat (page 104)

STATION 2

Mountain climber (page 156)

STATION 3

Single-arm dumbbell swing (page 143)

STATION 4

T-pushup (page 11)

STATION 5

Split squat (page 106)

STATION 6

Dumbbell row (page 34)

STATION 7

Dumbbell side lunge and touch (page 113)

STATION 8

Pushup position row (page 13)

For the pushup position row, refer to the pushup and row on page 13. Simply do the row portion of the exercise, without the pushup.

STATION 9

Dumbbell lunge and rotation (page 111)

STATION 10

Dumbbell push press (page 60)

WORKOUT LOG

DATE: **TODAY'S WEIGHT:**

EXERCISE	SETS	REPS	TIME	WEIGHT	NOTES

DATE: **TODAY'S WEIGHT:**

EXERCISE	SETS	REPS	TIME	WEIGHT	NOTES

Photocopy these pages so you can follow along at the gym.

DATE: **TODAY'S WEIGHT:**

EXERCISE	SETS	REPS	TIME	WEIGHT	NOTES

DATE: **TODAY'S WEIGHT:**

EXERCISE	SETS	REPS	TIME	WEIGHT	NOTES

FOOD LOG

DATE:

FOOD/DRINK	CALORIES
Breakfast	
Snack	
Lunch	
Snack	
Dinner	
Snack	
Total for the Day	
Did you drink at least 8 glasses of water? ___Y ___N	
Notes:	

DATE:

FOOD/DRINK	CALORIES
Breakfast	
Snack	
Lunch	
Snack	
Dinner	
Snack	
Total for the Day	
Did you drink at least 8 glasses of water? ___Y ___N	
Notes:	

DATE:

FOOD/DRINK	CALORIES
Breakfast	
Snack	
Lunch	
Snack	
Dinner	
Snack	
Total for the Day	
Did you drink at least 8 glasses of water? ___Y ___N	
Notes:	

DATE:

FOOD/DRINK	CALORIES
Breakfast	
Snack	
Lunch	
Snack	
Dinner	
Snack	
Total for the Day	
Did you drink at least 8 glasses of water? ___Y ___N	
Notes:	

FOOD LOG

DATE:

FOOD/DRINK	CALORIES
Breakfast	
Snack	
Lunch	
Snack	
Dinner	
Snack	
Total for the Day	
Did you drink at least 8 glasses of water? ___Y ___N	
Notes:	

DATE:

FOOD/DRINK	CALORIES
Breakfast	
Snack	
Lunch	
Snack	
Dinner	
Snack	
Total for the Day	
Did you drink at least 8 glasses of water? ___Y ___N	
Notes:	